— THE —
HANDMADE
mama

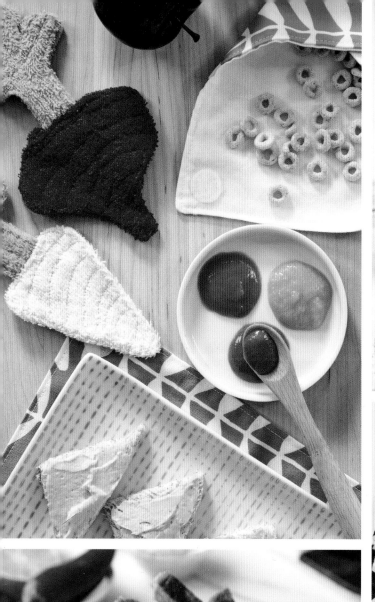

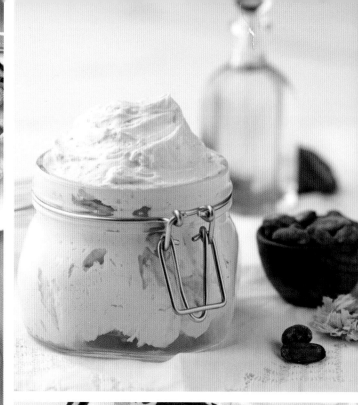

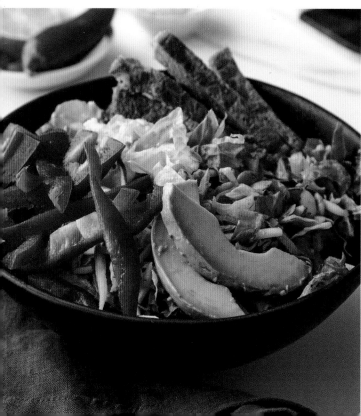

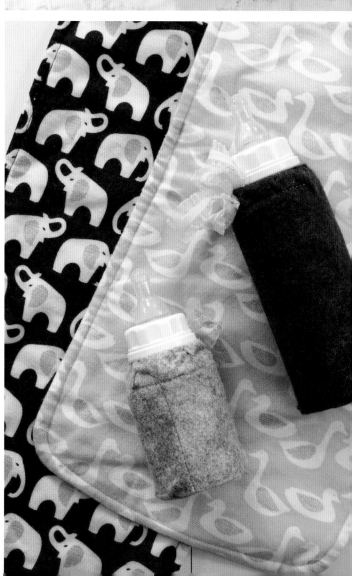

— THE —
HANDMADE
mama

**SIMPLE CRAFTS, HEALTHY RECIPES, AND NATURAL
BATH + BODY PRODUCTS FOR MAMA AND BABY**

MARY HELEN LEONARD

photography by
KIMBERLY DAVIS

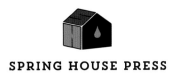

SPRING HOUSE PRESS

Publisher: Paul McGahren
Editorial Director: Matthew Teague
Editor: Kerri Grzybicki
Design: Lindsay Hess
Layout: Jodie Delohery
Illustration: Mary Helen Leonard
Photography: Kimberly Davis

Spring House Press
P.O. Box 239
Whites Creek, TN 37189

ISBN: 978-1-940611-71-6

Library of Congress Control Number: 2018935271

Printed in the United States of America

10 9 8 7 6 5 4 3 2 1

Note: The following list contains names used in *The Handmade Mama* that may be registered with the United States Copyright Office: American Academy of Pediatrics; American Felt and Craft; Baby Boot Camp; Baby Earth; Bee Well Pediatrics; Birch Organic Fabrics; Bob's Red Mill; Campaign for Safe Cosmetics; Care Calendar; Celebration Nutrition; City Moms Blog Network; Columbia University; Consumer Safety; Cookistry; Cookistry Reviews; Cool Mom Eats; Cool Mom Picks; DEET; Eco-PUL; Elephant Journal; Environmental Working Group; Etsy; Facebook; Fit 4 Mom; Fluff Love University; Fred Rogers; From Nature with Love; Granny Smith; Great Moments in Parenting; Hello Glow; Hike It Baby; Hilah Cooking; Honey Be Good Fabric; Honeycrisp; How to Talk So Kids Will Listen; India Tree; International Board-Certified Lactation Consultant ; International Federation of Professional Aromatherapists; International Lactation Consultant Association; Jennifer Pierce Health; Kelly Mom; La Leche League; Lemon Tree Supplies; *Make Ahead Bread; Make It Easy: 120 Mix-and-Match Recipes to Cook from Scratch—with Smart Store-Bought Shortcuts When You Need Them;* Mama Natural; Mary Makes Good; mason jar; Meal Train; Meetup; Mighty Nest; Mommypotamus; Mother Rising; Mountain Rose Herbs; Munching on Books; Natural Beauty Workshop; Nutella; Organic Consumer's Association; Organic Cotton Plus; ParentAbility; Picardin; Scary Mommy; *Seinfeld;* Spoonflower; Sriracha; The National Association for Holistic Aromatherapy; The Natural Baby Company; Thought Catalog; Velcro; Vermont Soap; Wellness Mama; While She Naps; YogaDork.

The information in this book is given in good faith; however, no warranty is given, nor are results guaranteed. Your safety is your responsibility. Neither Spring House Press nor the author assume any responsibility for any injuries or accidents.

To learn more about Spring House Press books, or to find a retailer near you, email info@springhousepress.com or visit us at www.springhousepress.com.

acknowledgements

This was a very hard book to write. I've always been a fairly confident person when it came to my own knowledge and creativity, but parenthood has been a humbling experience. I knew from the start of this project that I was no parenting expert, and at times that made finding the courage to share tips from my own experience quite difficult.

As I researched parts of the book, I learned a lot—but not nearly as much as I've learned firsthand settling into life as a mother. The biggest truth I've come to is that all moms are different; all families are different; all babies are different. As such, there is hardly ever one "right" answer to any parenting question. I'm thankful to all the wise and wonderful parents in my life for sharing their experiences with me. It helped a lot.

I started this project in the afterglow of having my first child, and while I was utterly exhausted, I was happier than I had ever been in my life. Shortly after my son's first birthday I got pregnant, and almost three months later, lost the baby. I was heartbroken, of course, and wondered how I would ever write a whole book on baby care.

With time, patience, and the loving support of my family, I was able to get back to work, and with a generous extension granted by the publisher, felt like I could perhaps pull the project off after all. During the course of writing, our family suffered four more pregnancy losses—including the loss of a twin during my most recent pregnancy. All in all, it has taken almost two years to write this book. I want to thank my editor, Matthew Teague, and my agent, Sally Ekus, for their kindness, patience, and understanding during what was an incredibly painful time in my personal life.

I have to say some special words of thanks: To my sister Heather, for providing editing and feedback every step of the way. To my Mom, for testing out recipes and sewing patterns, and, of course, for teaching me to sew in the first place. And a big thanks to everyone who took on toddler-wrangling duty so I could bury myself in writing a book (my husband Scott, my parents, and my sister Sarah).

I also want to thank the many fabulous contributors who provided recipes, projects, and words of wisdom. Hilah Johnson, Donna Currie, Sarah Kamalsky, Tanja Knutson, Stephanie Darby, Stacie Billis, Dr. Suzanne Van Benthuysen, Sara Kleinsmith, and Jennifer Pierce, I'm thrilled you are all a part of this book. Last but not least, a huge thank you to everyone who has read my blog, bought my first book, and shared my work. This would not be possible without your support.

contents

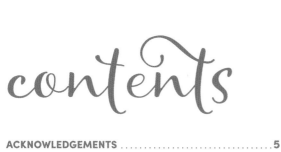
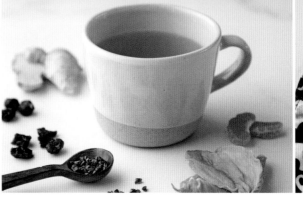
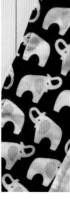

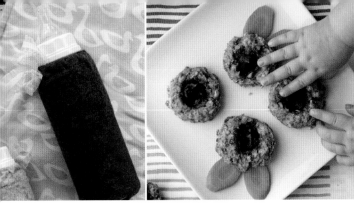
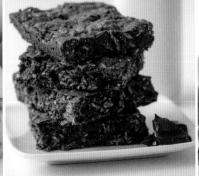
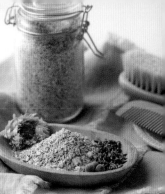

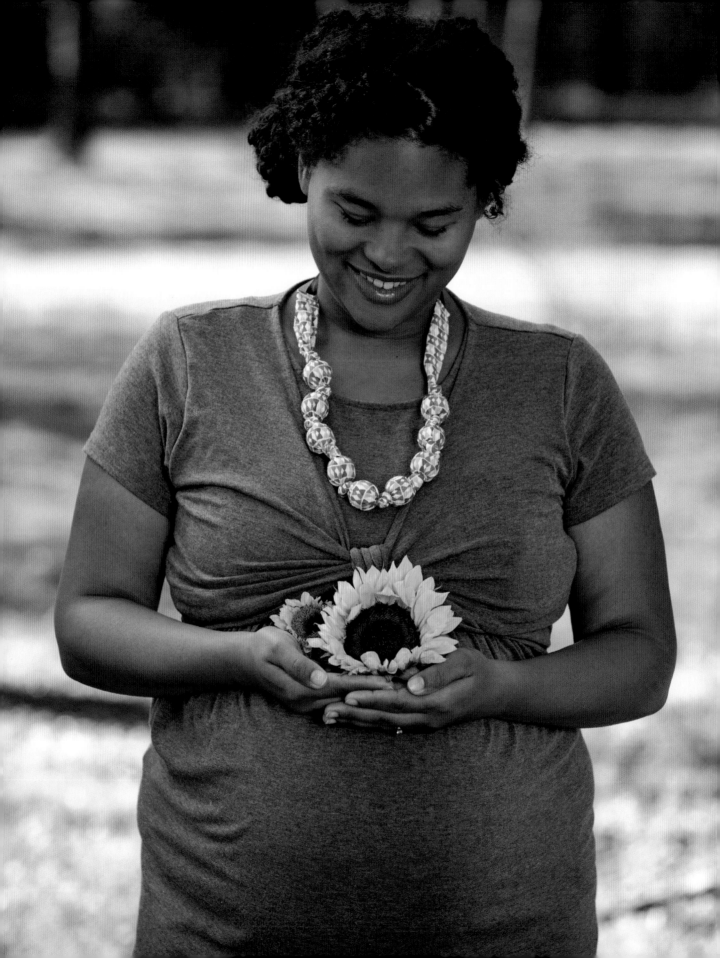

MAMAHOOD

ma·ma·hood

[ˈmäməˌho͝od/]

noun: The state of being a mama.

A lot of cliches are thrown around when people talk about becoming parents. Expecting mothers and fathers are often showered with a strange blend of congratulations and vague warnings as they deliver the news to friends and family. People tell you that everything will change, that your life will never be the same—in many ways, they are correct.

Becoming a parent is one of the single most life-altering experiences many people will ever have, and like any transformation, it doesn't always come easy. From pregnancy to birth and for years beyond, a parent's life is peppered with challenges, sacrifice, and sometimes even physical pain—but it is also infused with a sense of joy and satisfaction that somehow makes everything worthwhile.

To devote oneself to another in such a way, to experience the bliss of unconditional love, and to watch the creature who you nurture blossom into someone you love more with every passing day is more than transformative. Simply put, it makes life worth living.

From the moment you feel that spark of love in your heart that sets you on the path to finding your baby, you are a mama, and you always will be. Welcome to mamahood, beautiful sister. It's good over here. ➡

why go handmade?

A HEALTHY START

Making your own food, skin care products, and everyday objects allows you to choose exactly what you put on and into your body. While the popularity of green and natural products is on the rise, and it is becoming easier to find natural store-bought items, these are often expensive, and sifting through the brands to find products that are truly as healthful as advertised can be an exhausting process. Many of the everyday products we rely on through pregnancy and baby's first year are actually quite simple to make at home, giving mama and baby a safe and natural alternative to the confusing and sometimes even toxic big-box baby industry.

CONSUMER WASTE AND THE NEXT GENERATION

When you consider the fact that plastic didn't become an everyday material until around the 1940s, it's fairly astounding to see how much plastic waste has been accumulated in our landfills, oceans, and wilderness. Unfortunately, our society's dependence on nonbiodegradable materials like plastic doesn't seem to be slowing down anytime soon.

Typical families are buying and discarding things like toys, clothes, and baby gear every day. Tossing out a cracked plastic sippy cup may not seem like a big deal, but when you consider the resources consumed and carbon emissions created just to make that cup, it hurts a little.

Creating and cherishing handmade items and using sustainable materials is one small thing that you can do to avoid consumer waste and inspire the next generation to make better decisions when it comes to our environment.

CUSTOMIZE SOLUTIONS TO YOUR FAMILY NEEDS

Sure, you could spend hours scouring the Internet for a snack pouch in your child's favorite color or a diaper cream that only contains the specific ingredients you've deemed hiney-worthy, or you could spend that time making it with your own two hands. You pick the color. You choose the ingredients. You make adjustments to suit your own tastes and needs. There's nothing better than custom-made, and when you do it yourself, it can actually be affordable!

THE VALUE OF PRACTICAL ART

As a busy working parent, I base many of my buying decisions on practicality. Which item will last the longest? Which costs loss? How bad is it for us? These are the questions I tend to ask while shopping for necessities. Rarely do I have the luxury of picking the object that speaks to me on an artistic level; yet, I've come to find that the presence of beautiful things in my everyday life gives me a sense of comfort and joy. Whether it's a handthrown coffee mug or a homemade quilt, that little touch of beauty can enrich our everyday experiences in a way that is hard to quantify. I find that handmade objects possess an inherent beauty, adding a unique value to the practice of making things yourself.

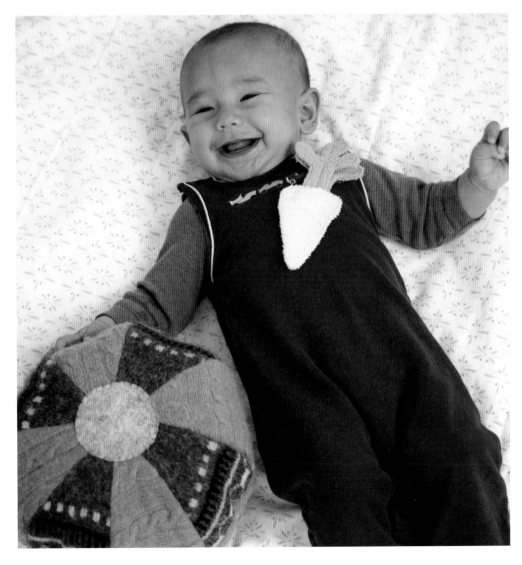

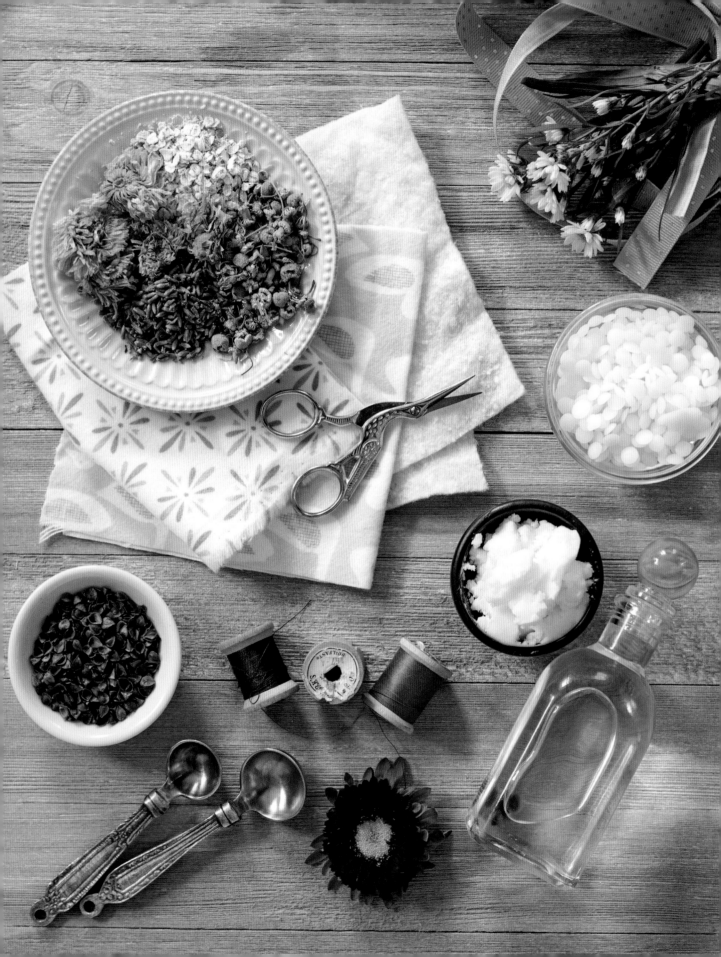

↓

chapter 1

MATERIALS & TECHNIQUES

When it comes to caring for mamas and babies, I like to keep things as simple as possible. That means choosing whole foods for cooking, natural ingredients for body care, and plant-based fabrics for sewing whenever possible. Of course, shortcuts and exceptions are a fact of life—all the more when one is juggling the many responsibilities of motherhood.

In this book, I like to recommend my favorite ingredients and materials for each project, but I also encourage you to embrace other solutions that work for you. If making all-purpose gluten-free flour from scratch seems like too much work, go ahead and buy a bag from the store. I love using wool and canvas to make my changing pads, but if you need something more resistant to liquids, give polyurethane laminate (PUL) diapering material a try.

Making your own food, body care products, and everyday objects can be a very rewarding endeavor! With a little practice, I think you'll find that the techniques used in this book are easy enough to make cooking, formulating, and even sewing a breeze. As you become familiar with natural ingredients and materials I hope that you'll gain the same deep appreciation I have for their wholesome nature and vast benefits. →

sewing tips & techniques

WHY GO NATURAL WITH FABRIC FOR BABY?

Conventional cotton is often farmed using extremely heavy loads of fertilizers and pesticides—two substances that cause major concerns for both human health and environmental well-being. Just like food or skin-care products, materials made from plants farmed with heavy pesticide may contain concerning residues. Just think about how much time we spend with our clothing or bedding touching our skin. Yuck! Since buying all organic clothing and bedding isn't always an affordable choice, I suggest picking your battles. An organic crib sheet, for example, is a small investment that you can feel good about.

TYPES OF FABRIC

There are many fabrics in the world to choose from, but my favorites for baby care and everyday use are found in this book. I tend to lean toward natural fabrics. Materials like cotton, hemp, and bamboo offer eco-friendly and sustainable options. They also tend to be more comfortable and durable than their synthetic alternatives. However, there are synthetic fabrics that can come in very handy for baby care, like polyurethane laminate (PUL) and microfleece.

Bamboo Fleece: This amazingly soft and absorbent fabric can help act as a moisture barrier, making it an excellent choice for breast pads, diaper liners, and washcloths.

Batting: Usually made from cotton, wool, or polyester, batting is a fluffy layer of material that helps to soften, fill, or insulate between two other layers of fabric. Quilts typically contain a layer of batting. This technique used to make quilts and blankets fluffy can also be used in other kinds of projects, like eye masks and moon pads.

Cotton Canvas: Canvas is a thick, durable material often used for utility items such as lunch bags, outdoor play mats, or tote bags.

Cotton Flannel: The soft, fuzzy texture of flannel makes it very popular for baby care, pillows, and softies. The material has a fairly thin texture, so it is also very easy to work with.

Denim: Like canvas, denim is a great choice for items that require extra durability. Its tight weave and thickness can also help repel moisture.

Jersey Knit: This soft, stretchy material is popular for use in clothing. You are probably most familiar with it in the form of a T-shirt. It makes a great choice for baby clothes, hats, and pajamas.

Microfleece: Though microfleece can be made from natural materials, synthetic microfleece is often less expensive and easier to find. Synthetic microfleece can be used in mama and baby projects, but it will lack the breathability and comfort of microfleece made from bamboo or other natural fibers.

Muslin: Muslin is a thin fabric often made from cotton. It comes in both white and natural colors and is usually used as a simple lining or backing.

Polyurethane Laminate (PUL): This synthetic material has a water-resistant coating that makes it an incredibly popular choice for cloth diaper covers, wet bags, and changing mats. For food projects, like snack bags or lunch boxes, look for Eco-PUL. Eco-PUL is a food-safe fabric, while regular PUL is not.

Quilter's Cotton: This thin, easy-to-use material (also referred to as calico) comes in an impressive variety of prints and colors and can be used for many everyday projects. Its most common use is for quilting, but this versatile fabric can also be used to make clothes, toys, or crafts.

Terrycloth: Terrycloth is a highly textured fabric used most commonly in washcloths and bath towels. It is highly absorbent and perfect for tubby time.

Terrycloth is typically made of cotton, but can also be made from other natural materials like hemp, bamboo, or flax.

Waxed Canvas: Waxed canvas is a food-safe water-resistant material used in lunch boxes, snack bags, and totes. It is available in a range of prints and colors. Waxed canvas resembles another common material called oilcloth, but these two fabrics are quite different; oilcloth is not considered to be food safe, and in some cases is not considered to be child safe either.

Wool Felt: Wool felt is a thick, fuzzy material that is somehow both soft and scratchy. This dense fabric makes an excellent moisture barrier for changing pads and diapers, but it is also a popular material for making toys, puppets, and home crafts.

PREPPING FABRICS

Brand-new fabric can sometimes shrink or change texture slightly after being laundered. This makes it important to prepare new fabrics by washing and drying them before use. This helps make sure that your projects will still look great after you put them through the wash. To prepare flannel, jersey, quilter's cotton, denim, canvas, or terrycloth, wash in cold water with a gentle detergent and dry with low heat. Iron if necessary, as folds and wrinkles can make fabric harder to work with. Delicate fabrics like wool or silk should be washed by hand with gentle detergent and air dried.

ASK AN *expert*

Q: Which materials do you like best when sewing for babies?

A: I am a big fan of cotton knit. Soft and stretchy, it feels good and keeps movement free and easy. Birch Organic Fabrics, in particular, hits it out of the park with a line of super-soft, baby-friendly fabrics in crazy-adorable prints. I mean, Charley Harper on fabric? Yes, please!

—*Sarah Kamalsky, SarahJayn.com*

NOTIONS

More than just a great idea, notions are what we call all the little bits and baubles that go along with sewing projects.

Bias Tape: Bias tape is a pre-cut and folded strip of fabric that can be used to add bindings to seams on blankets, clothing, and crafts. It is sold in a variety of colors at most fabric shops, but ambitious sewers can make their own from quilter's cotton or broadcloth.

Elastic: Elastic is basically a stretchy rubber band woven with knit material, and is used to provide stretch to clothing and crafts. Elastic comes in a variety of sizes and shapes, so be sure to find the specific type called for in your project.

Fiberfill: The fluffy stuffing packed into stuffed animals and cushions is fiberfill. The most common type of fiberfill is made from polyester, but recycled or natural alternatives are gaining popularity and becoming more widely available.

Hook-and-Loop Tape: You probably know this material best by the brand name of Velcro. Hook-and-loop tape is used to fasten clothing, seal bags, or make pretty much anything stick shut. Look for standard-backed hook-and-loop tape (as opposed to adhesive-backed) for sewing projects.

Sewing Needles: Whether you are working by hand or by machine, you can't sew without a needle. When hand sewing, look for a general-use needle. For machine sewing, my favorite all-around needle is a universal point in size 14/90. While a basic needle will get you a long way, projects tend to go easier and turn out better when using a needle that matches the material.

Snaps and Fasteners: There are lots of different notions used to fasten things shut. Some of the most commonly used devices include buttons, buckles, snaps, toggles, and hook and eye fasteners. Most of these items can be sewn on by hand, but sturdier adhesion is possible with tools like snap pliers.

Straight Pins and Safety Pins: Straight pins are essential for careful, meticulous sewing. These tiny, sharp little pieces of

SEWING NEEDLE CHART

NEEDLE TYPE	NEEDLE SIZE	FABRIC
Ballpoint	10/70, 12/80	Jersey knit, single knit
Ballpoint	14/90	Doubleknit, sweatshirt, sweater knit
Ballpoint, Universal	70/11, 75/11, 80/12	PUL
Denim/Jeans	16/100	Canvas, denim
Universal	14/90	Flannel, terrycloth, quilter's cotton
Universal	9/70, 11/80	Microfleece
Universal	16/100, 18/100	Wool felt
Universal	100/16, 110/18	Waxed canvas

THREAD INFORMATION

THREAD MATERIAL	THREAD WEIGHT	FABRIC
Cotton	All-purpose	Flannel, terrycloth, quilter's cotton
Cotton, Polyester	All-purpose	Microfleece, PUL, wool felt
Polyester	All-purpose	Doubleknit, knit jersey, sweatshirt, sweater knit
Cotton, Polyester	Heavy, denim	Canvas, denim, waxed canvas

wire are sharp on one end and flat or capped on the other. Their job is to hold fabric together as it is sewn. It's a good idea to have a tidy little supply of pins handy as you sew, ideally located in an adorable pin cushion. Safety pins are capped pins that remain in place even as the project is jostled around. These are great for quilting, turning out projects, and securing particularly tricky sewing projects.

Thread: An all-purpose weight cotton or polyester thread will work for most projects in this book. However, taking the time to make sure you are using the best thread for the job can help sewing go more smoothly and ensure that the final product will be both sturdy and beautiful.

HOW TO USE THE PATTERNS IN THIS BOOK

The patterns in this book are all fairly simple and suitable for beginner to intermediate sewers. Patterns for the projects in this book are located on page 188. Several of the projects in this book do not include patterns. These projects have measurements for cutting included in the tutorial instructions. Unless otherwise

noted, all patterns use a ¼-inch (6mm) seam allowance.

STARTING AND FINISHING A SEAM

Whenever you begin a new seam it is important to start and finish that seam to secure it. Otherwise, it can unravel. To start your seam, make your first stitches, then put the sewing machine in reverse and stitch back over what you've sewed so far (this is called a backstitch—how appropriate!). Set the machine back to forward, sew over those stitches, and continue the rest of your seam. Finish the seam using the same method of backstitching over those stitches to secure them.

BASIC MACHINE STITCHES

While most sewing machines these days come with a dizzying array of fanciful stitches, you typically will only need a handful for everyday sewing. In this book, we only use two!

Straight Stitch: This is your machine's most basic everyday stitch. It goes forward and backward in a line as straight as you can steer it. Unless otherwise noted, this is the stitch you will

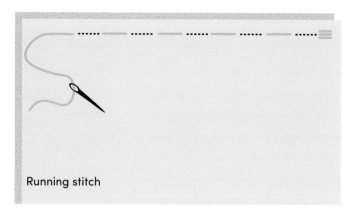

Running stitch

use in every project in this book. Your machine will probably allow you to adjust the length of this stitch. In general, you'll want to use a shorter length for thinner fabrics and more detailed stitching (sewing curves, for example) and a longer stitch for thicker fabrics and less detailed stitching (like quilting a play mat).

Zigzag Stitch: Mastering the zigzag stitch instantly kicks a beginning sewer up a notch. This versatile stitch can help you tidy up seams to discourage fraying, applique layers of fabric together, or just add a cute detail to projects. You should be able to adjust both the width and the length of this stitch, going from a wide geometric pattern to a smooth, tight satin stitch like you'd see in embroidery. I recommend test-driving this stitch on scrap fabric before using it in a project. In fact, I use a scrap of fabric to get my length and width just right every time I use the zigzag stitch.

HAND SEWING

Sewing machines are fantastic inventions, but there are still many times when a few stitches of hand sewing are necessary. One thing I've learned through a lifetime of sewing is that the smaller and finer you can make your stitches, the neater the final product will be. There is a wonderful art to hand sewing and though it can involve many kinds of marvelous specialty stitches, I really only use three on a regular basis.

Running Stitch: This is a very basic stitch for hand sewing that mimics the straight stitch a sewing machine makes.

1. Thread your needle with a generous portion of cut thread. Pin the two pieces of fabric together, then push the needle through both. Pull the needle out until only a short tail remains, then repeat that stitch over itself two times to anchor the thread. Think of this as the manual version of a backstitch.

2. Weave the needle in and out of fabric in 1/8 to 1/4-inch (3 to 6mm) stitches.

3. To finish, repeat the last stitch over itself two times, pulling the thread snugly. Snip excess thread.

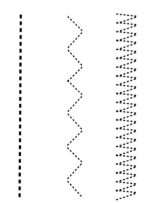

Straight stitch   Zigzag stitch

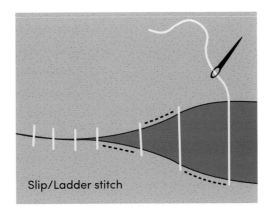

Slip/Ladder stitch

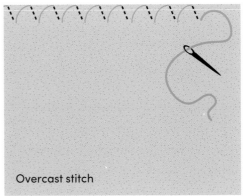

Overcast stitch

Slip/Ladder Stitch: This stitch is used to form a (mostly) invisible seam between two pieces of fabric. It is perfect for finishing up items that you have turned out, like the ribbon softies (page 175) or buckwheat pillows (page 53) in this book.

1. Thread your needle with a generous portion of cut thread. Open the two pieces of fabric and sink your needle into a piece of the finished seam's raw edge.

2. Pull the thread through until only a short tail is left, then pull it through two more times to secure it. Push the needle through the top of the fabric just before the opening begins.

3. Fold (and pin if possible) the two pieces of fabric in toward each other, mimicking the look of a finished seam.

4. Push the needle into one side of the folded fabric and out directly across the fold, stitching across and beneath the fabric. Move down the fold just a little and repeat the stitch.

5. Continue moving down and stitching across the fold until the opening is completely closed. To finish, repeat the last stitch over itself two times, pulling the thread snug. Snip off excess thread.

Overcast Stitch: The overcast stitch, or whipstitch, helps tack down wild edges and keeps loose fabrics from fraying. It's a great choice for stitching felt shapes onto fabric, sewing patches on a stuffed animal, or adding a simple binding to a no-sew project.

1. Thread your needle with a generous portion of cut thread. Pin the two pieces of fabric together, then push the needle through both. Pull the needle out until only a short tail remains, then repeat that stitch over itself two times to anchor the thread.

2. Make a diagonal stitch that loops over the edge of the fabric and repeat that stitch down the length of the fabric edge. Space the stitches according to your preference.

3. To finish, repeat the last stitch over itself two times, pulling the thread snugly. Snip excess thread.

TURNING OUT

If you take a close look at your clothes, you'll notice that the edges of seams are usually hidden inside garments. This little magic trick is often accomplished by sewing the item inside-out. When the majority of sewing is finished, the item will need to be turned right-side out again. If you are working on something large, like a shirt, this is as easy as can be. If you are working with something smaller or more complicated, like a stuffed animal or a long cord, the process can be a bit more tricky. These are my two favorite techniques for turning out tricky bits of fabric.

Safety Pin: This method works especially well for long, rectangular pieces, such as cords, belts, or tubes. Fasten a large safety pin to one end of the inside-out tube, then push it through the middle until it comes out the other side. You can then roll the remaining fabric until the entire piece is right-side out.

Chopstick: I love chopsticks for turning out tiny or oddly shaped pieces. One end of the stick is thicker than the other, giving you two different shapes to poke around with. The key to using a chopstick to turn out fabric is moving gently and having patience. You don't want to push so hard that you rip through the fabric. Take your time, but be thorough and make sure to turn out every little fold with care.

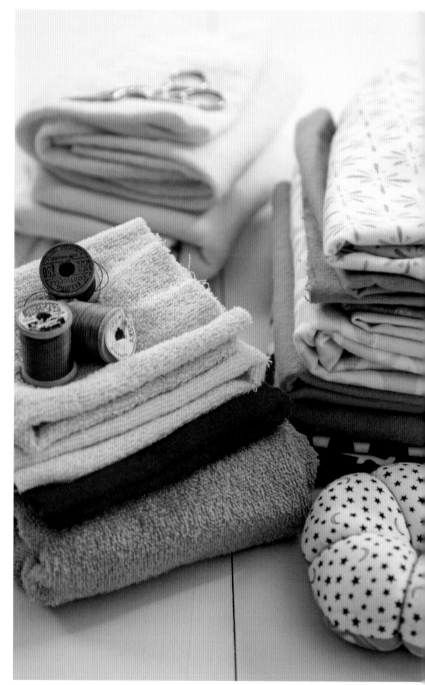

bath & body tips & techniques

WHY GO NATURAL WITH BATH & BODY FOR BABY?

Babies really don't need much in the way of bath and body products. A little natural soap and water goes a long way. A touch of apricot kernel oil or mango butter is just enough to keep their skin moisturized and happy. So why are commercial baby products usually packed with artificial fragrances and colors? Babies smell sweet enough on their own, and synthetic additives come with a laundry list of possible health concerns that just don't seem to be worth the risk. Save your money and your peace of mind by sticking to a simple, handmade natural bath and body routine for your wee one instead.

LESS IS MORE

Bath and body products tend to have very long ingredient lists, but really, we only need a few healthy ingredients to keep our skin and hair happy. Using simple handmade products allows you complete control over what goes on your body. By making these basic products at home you won't have to worry about synthetic preservatives, fragrances, or additives that have questionable reputations when it comes to health.

FRESH IS BEST

One drawback to making your own products is that they don't often have the super-long shelf lives we've grown accustomed to with commercial products. This means you'll need to make small batches of product and use them quickly in order to avoid spoilage. Most of the recipes in this book will last for at least three months unless otherwise noted.

DRIED HERBS

Dried herbs allow us to add special botanical benefits to homemade products in a gentle way. Unlike essential oils, dried herbs add their benefit at a very low potency. This often makes them a safer and more cautious choice for homemade mama and baby products.

Calendula: A type of dried marigold petal, calendula has long been used in herbal medicines for its healing and soothing benefits.

Chamomile: Tiny chamomile flowers are prized for their anti-inflammatory properties. This makes them ideal for soothing dry, itchy, or irritated skin.

Lavender: A quintessential herb for use in bath and body care, lavender not only smells wonderful, it may also help to soothe, heal, and cleanse when added to herbal recipes.

Plantain Leaf: In herbal medicine, this dried herb is believed to help reduce pain and swelling.

Vanilla Bean: The comforting scent of vanilla is added to recipes for the pure pleasure of it. I've found that its aroma blends well with almost any combination of herbs or ingredients.

FOOD INGREDIENTS

Apple Cider Vinegar: When properly diluted, apple cider vinegar helps to balance skin's pH, tame troublesome bacteria, and soothe itchy, irritated skin. It is an essential part of any natural hair care routine, and acts as both a conditioner and detangler. Buy raw, organic, and unfiltered apple cider vinegar when you can, as this will be, by far, the most potent type available.

Oat Starch: Starch is used to add softness and silkiness to the feel of many skin care products.

Whole Oats: The soothing benefit of oatmeal is well-known in folk medicine. Using whole oats allows us to also make use of this ingredient's gentle exfoliation.

OTHER INGREDIENTS

Arrowroot Powder: This dried and powdered herbal product adds a silky slip to powders, lotions, and milk baths.

Kaolin Clay: Also known as China clay, kaolin clay is one of the most gentle cosmetic clays available. Unlike many other types of cosmetic clay, kaolin is not overly drying to the skin, making it a superb choice for mama and baby care.

Liquid Castile Soap: This versatile natural soap can be used for everything from shampoo to dish soap. It is truly an all-purpose wonder and usually made with just a handful of ingredients. Liquid castile has a thinner consistency than most commercial soaps, but it does not lack potency. In fact, it can be diluted with water, herbal tea, or aloe vera to make a quick body wash or foaming soap.

Zinc Oxide: Traditionally used in a variety of ointments, you may recognize the bright white color of zinc oxide from sunscreen and diaper creams. Used to soothe skin and speed healing, zinc makes an excellent additive to diapering recipes.

VEGETABLE OILS

Also commonly referred to as carrier oils or nourishing oils, vegetable oils are usually pressed from the seeds or nuts of a plant. Look for virgin, cold-pressed, and organic varieties to find the highest quality oils with the most potent benefits. These oils can be used as-is to moisturize skin and hair, for massage, or incorporated into bath and body recipes.

Apricot Kernel Oil: This light and moisturizing oil is extremely versatile. It is an affordable, easy-to-find choice for almost every homemade bath and body product, so I buy it in pretty big bottles!

Avocado Oil: Avocado oil has a thicker, heavier texture than apricot kernel oil, so it's great for recipes that need a little extra conditioning power, like belly butter.

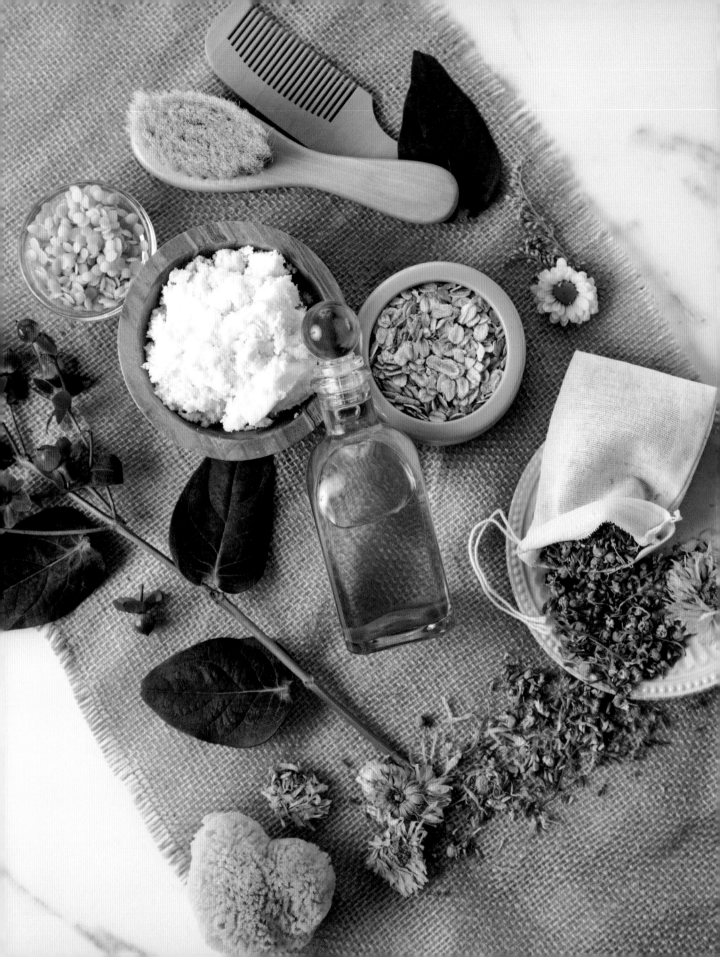

Argan Oil: Argan oil is packed with vitamin E, fatty acids, and antioxidants that can help skin stay soft and elastic as it grows. It can be a bit pricey, so I only use a little bit in my most special recipes. Look for 100% pure virgin argan oil so you aren't paying for a diluted version.

Castor Oil: This super-sticky and greasy carrier oil helps form a barrier between the skin and outside moisture.

VEGETABLE BUTTERS

Vegetable butters are far thicker and heavier than carrier oils, and are used to add rich conditioning benefits to body and skin care recipes. These rich butters can also be used as-is on dry skin as intensive moisturizers.

Cocoa Butter: Pure cocoa butter has a characteristic aroma that you will instantly recognize as the rich, creamy chocolate of your dreams. This super-hard butter is an intense conditioner—perfect for helping skin stay supple and elastic.

Cupuacu Butter: A treat from the Amazon, cupuacu butter has a texture and moisturizing quality similar to shea butter. This makes it a great alternative for people with latex sensitivities, as they can sometime find shea butter to be irritating.

Mango Butter: Mango butter is a wonderful choice for baby care because it agrees with almost every skin type and rarely causes irritation. Its texture is a bit lighter and softer than shea or cocoa butter, but it still moisturizes quite nicely.

Shea Butter: This classic beauty ingredient comes in several varieties. Raw shea is touted as the most effective, but it has a strong nutty aroma. Refined shea butter is nearly odorless and colorless, and tends to be easier to work with than raw shea.

WAXES

Wax is used to harden balms and body butters.

Beeswax: Beeswax is the most common and easiest wax to use, having a relatively soft and pliable texture. Look for natural cosmetic-grade beeswax. This wax is naturally golden or yellow in color but is also available in a white variety that has been bleached with light.

Candelilla Wax: This plant-based wax is a good choice for vegans, or those who prefer not to use animal-based ingredients. It has a much harder texture, so you'll need to add just a pinch less of wax when working with candelilla.

BASIC EQUIPMENT & SUPPLIES

Double Boiler: These specialty pots allow you to melt fragile ingredients, like vegetable butters and waxes, using indirect heat. They are also great for warming oil or water to make infusions. If you don't want to invest in a double boiler, try placing a stainless-steel bowl over a pot of hot water or placing a large mason jar into a pot with 1 to 2 inches of simmering water. Just be careful!

Electric Mixer with Whisk Attachment: Whether you use a handheld mixer or a stand mixer, you will appreciate the extra help when making whipped body butters. Mixers are also quite handy for baking!

Empty Bottles and Jars: You can find most of the packaging items you'll need at the grocery store. Mason jars come in almost every shape and size you need for baby and mama care, and plastic squeeze bottles are usually easy to find. Specialty items, like plastic bottles, foaming soap bottles, and powder shakers can be ordered online, or they can be saved, cleaned out, and re-used from commercial products.

Kitchen Scale: While you usually can get away with measuring spoons and cups, I find a kitchen scale to be much more accurate and consistent for making body care products at home.

---

handmade mama tip

PARABENS

Paraben-based preservatives help to keep commercially produced bath and body products stable on the shelf for long periods of time. In recent years, concern over the safety of these ingredients has been on the rise as possible links have been discovered between paraben use and skin irritation, hormone disruption, and cancer.

HOW TO APPROACH HOME REMEDIES

I like to think of myself as a fairly crunchy mama, but when it comes to home remedies and natural medicines, I tend to approach them with a healthy level of skepticism. This isn't because I prefer conventional medicine or pharmaceuticals. In fact, I fully support trying a natural and gentle solution as a first choice. My years in the natural living industry have granted me a deep respect for the power of herbs and natural medicines, which is exactly why I know they must be used with care.

I've also learned that botanical substances like herbs and essential oils can be extremely potent, and can carry serious side effects and contraindications. This holds especially true when it comes to treating babies and kids. Their tiny systems don't always process substances the way that adults do, and they can easily be overdosed, leading to serious illness and injury. Before trying out any herbal remedy, I urge you to first clear that remedy with your pediatrician.

There are plenty of tried-and-true home remedies that can be really helpful for babies, kids, and expecting mamas, but it's crucial that they be administered safely. Remember, just because something is natural, doesn't mean it's safe.

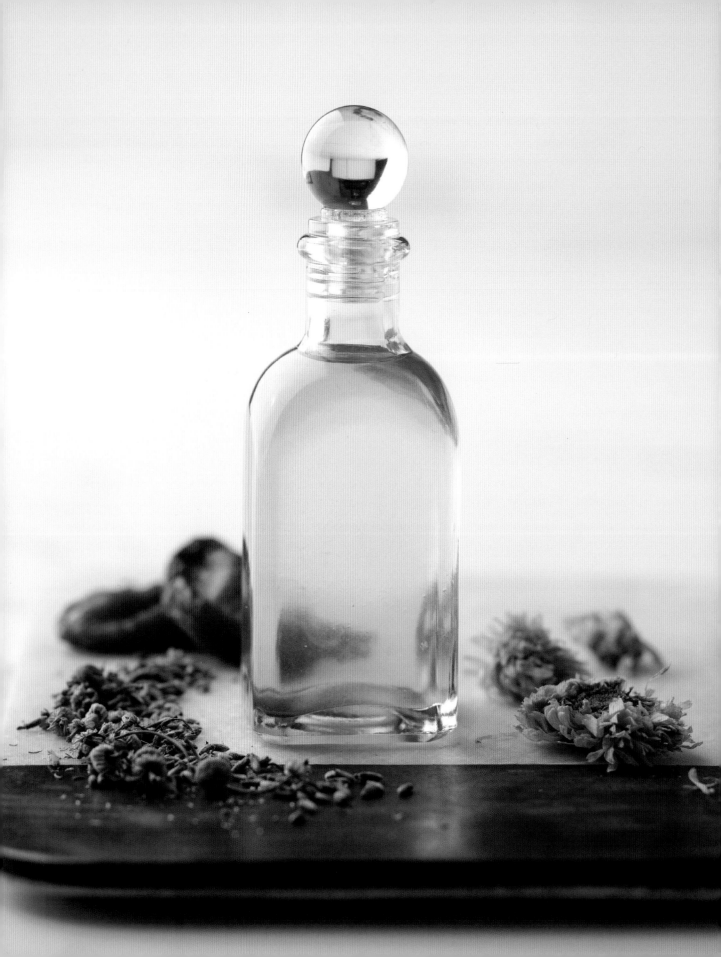

HERBAL BODY OIL

YIELD: *8 ounces (240 ml)*

O f all the recipes in this book, this one is my favorite by far. In our house we call this stuff Magic Oil. We use it for bedtime massage, to soothe dry or irritated skin from head to toe, and even as a hair conditioner when our tresses are feeling a bit too crispy.

This super-versatile oil also serves as a base ingredient for more advanced skin care recipes like balms, body butters, and diaper ointments. Infused with a blend of soothing herbs and sweet-smelling vanilla bean, this moisturizing oil really can feel magical as it makes rashes, dry skin, and even frowns disappear.

INGREDIENTS

- ½ vanilla bean
- 8 ounces (240 ml) apricot kernel oil
- 2 tablespoons (4 g) dried lavender buds
- 2 tablespoons (4 g) dried chamomile
- ¼ cup (4 g) dried calendula

DIRECTIONS

1. Using a small paring knife, split the vanilla bean open by slicing it down the middle.

2. Combine the vanilla bean, apricot kernel oil, lavender, chamomile, and calendula in a double boiler over medium heat for 60 minutes.

3. Remove the mixture from the heat and let cool for 30 minutes.

4. Strain the oil through fine mesh, cheesecloth, or a nut milk bag (used to strain solids out of homemade nut milk). Discard solids and store the infused oil in a bottle or jar at room temperature for up to 6 months.

TO USE

The oil can be applied directly to the skin as a body oil or massage oil. It can also be dabbed onto hair to serve as a leave-in conditioner or used as an ingredient in other recipes.

kitchen tips & techniques

WHY GO NATURAL FOR FEEDING MOM & BABY?

Growing a baby is hard work. From the moment of conception to the day your child graduates high school (and often for years to come), parents do their best to keep kids safe, happy, and healthy. A huge part of that job is making sure that mom and baby get plenty of nutrition from the very start. Being mindful of what we eat allows us to make the most of every bite. Once you start learning about what goes into making food, you will soon discover that, like so many things, less is more. Overly processed foods often contain more salt, sugar, and unhealthy additives than we should be consuming. Sticking to whole natural foods is a simple strategy for a lifetime of better health.

FEEDING MAMA

The typical symptoms and the additional nutritional needs of pregnancy present a bit of a challenge for many women. Your body needs a steady diet of healthy food, but our bodies don't always cooperate. Fierce cravings, aversions, and bouts of nausea can make eating well a difficult task to accomplish. After baby arrives, our body still has plenty of work to do healing itself and caring for baby. Still, many women are simply too tired or busy to make eating well a priority. Since you may not be able to eat as often or as much as

you'd like, making sure the food you do consume is dense in nutrients can be a big help. For me, the trick to a nutritious pregnancy and postpartum period was creating goals for myself each day. Instead of focusing on what not to eat, I chose to prioritize key foods like protein, leafy greens, healthy fats, and vegetables. The mama recipes in this book are those that I leaned on heavily before and after having my son.

FEEDING BABY

Feeding baby can be a real adventure, and a feat that is sometimes easier said than done. Setting goals for what you'd like baby's first year of feeding to look like is a healthy and proactive way to get started. If you choose to breast-feed, make sure to get plenty of education and support before baby arrives. Think about when and how you plan on introducing things like formula and solid foods. As you get to know your child and yourself in your role of mama, you may end up needing to adjust the goals you have set, but having a plan and a support system in place will help give those goals a fighting chance and provide you with the tools you need to tackle challenges along the way.

BASIC KITCHEN EQUIPMENT

Baby Dishes and Utensils: If going green is a priority for your family, you'll be thrilled to know that sustainable baby basics are becoming more and more easy to find. Look for products made from bamboo, stainless steel, silicone, and tempered glass.

Blender or Food Processor: A high-powered blender or food processor can be a real boon to the handmade mama. You'll need one or the other to make purees, fruit butters, smoothies, and other chopped, diced, or liquified foods.

Food Mill: A true wonder of kitchen technology, the food mill is a hand-operated device that pushes soft foods through a fine strainer while separating harder sections like peels, seeds, and stems.

Steamer Pot: Steaming is a quick and easy way to prepare simple fruits and veggies for purees and baby recipes. You can slide a steamer insert into a large saucepan with a tight-fitting lid, or purchase a steamer pot made exclusively for this purpose.

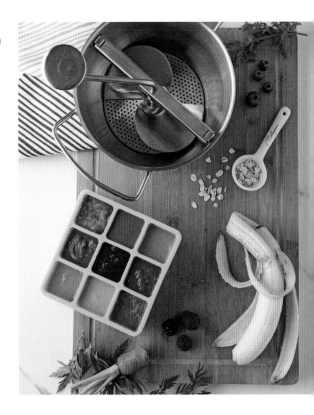

also crucial that babies and little kids be supervised as they eat.

PREPPING FINGER FOODS

When preparing food for babies and very young children, it is always important to keep their capabilities and limitations in mind. Certain foods, like grapes, are notorious choking hazards for wee ones. This is because their size and shape mimics the size and shape of a child's throat. Grapes should always be cut into small pieces (at least in halves or quarters) before being given to little ones. Keep that size and shape in mind while preparing bites and snacks like cookies, veggies, or fruits. For the same reason, it is

FREEZING & STORING BABY FOOD

Baby's first forays into solid food will involve shockingly small portions. Babies often start out with just one teaspoon or tablespoon of food at a time. Because making such a small amount of food is pretty much impossible, storing baby food becomes a big part of the baby-feeding process. Green mamas will prefer using glass storage containers, like screw-top jars, to store small portions of baby food. Silicone ice cube trays are also great for storing individual portions in the freezer. As a general rule, baby food lasts three to five days in the refrigerator or about three months in the freezer.

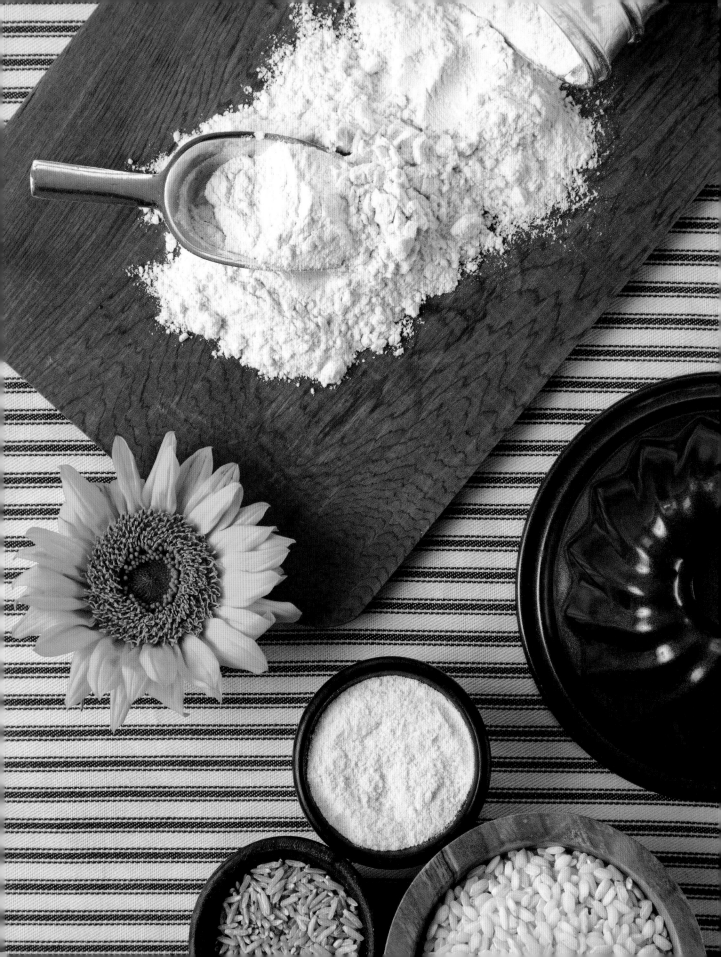

ALL-PURPOSE GLUTEN-FREE FLOUR

YIELD: *5 cups (1.2 L)*

If you plan on baking gluten-free recipes regularly, making your own all-purpose flour can save you a considerable amount of money. This flour works well for most basic recipes, such as muffins, cakes, and cookies. However, it does not do terribly well in traditional bread recipes. When using this flour as a substitute for general all-purpose or whole wheat flour, keep in mind that the product may require between 10 to 20% extra baking time.

INGREDIENTS

- 1 cup (240 ml) brown rice flour
- 1 cup (240 ml) potato starch
- 1 cup (240 ml) sweet rice flour
- 1 cup (240 ml) white rice flour
- 1 tablespoon plus 1 teaspoon (35 ml) xanthan gum

DIRECTIONS

1. Whisk ingredients together until thoroughly blended.
2. Store in airtight container for up to 6 months.

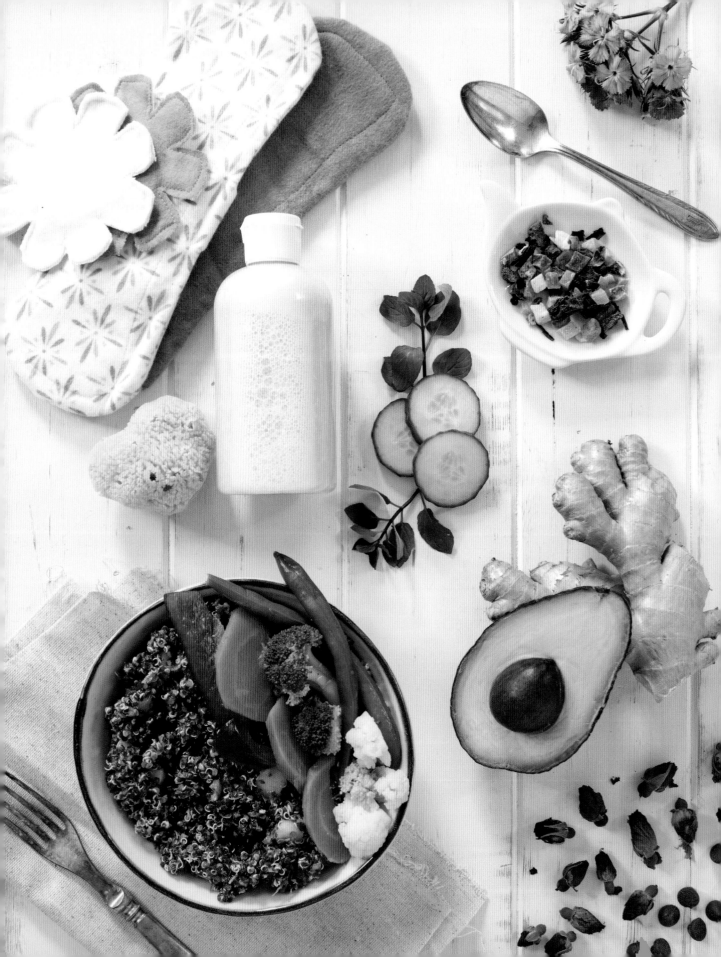

chapter 2

RECIPES & PROJECTS FOR MAMA

You are the perfect mama for this baby. Even more apparent than the words "jumbo shrimp," the phrase "perfect parent" is the ultimate oxymoron. We all have our moments of greatness and our unavoidable faults, and since parenthood is an experience that can leave even the greatest among us feeling naked and vulnerable, most moms and dads would have to admit that "perfect" just isn't an attainable goal when it comes to raising children.

Despite this, I do cling to the rosy-colored belief that even with my (cough, cough) *many* shortcomings, I am a perfect parent just as I am. And so, my dear friend, are you! If you can entertain the notion that God, or fate, or whatever you may like to see as destiny, placed this very specific soul in your care, than you'll see my point.

You are meant to be this baby's mother. Not some other, more perfect version of you. Just you—flaws and all. I think back on life with my own parents, two people who couldn't be more real if they tried, and I know that it isn't just their strengths who made me who I am today. I grew up watching them struggle as well as succeed. We loved each other. We fought each other. We lived together and saw each other laid bare as the perfectly imperfect people we were. They helped me become the woman I am today, and that's a person I have grown to take pride in. While it isn't always as simple as this sounds, you are meant to be this baby's mama. So as you begin your journey as a parent, try to remember to start this relationship off like any other. Relax. Take heart, and just be yourself. →

body care for mama

The transformation of your body during and after pregnancy is an amazing thing to watch. Treat yourself gently by creating your own personalized and natural bath and body products, and be mindful of the changes you're undergoing. As your baby grows, take the time to think through what will happen during the delivery and after you get your baby home. With some preparation, the postpartum transition is easier to manage.

BIRTH MANTRAS

Some of the best advice that I foolishly ignored before having my son came from a midwife during our birth class. She encouraged all of us to pick a birth mantra—a short phrase that we could repeat (either out loud or in our minds) during labor. The purpose of a birth mantra is to help mama focus, set her intentions, and remind her that she is strong, courageous, or simply that this, too, shall pass.

When our midwife asked the class for suggestions all I could think of was "Serenity Now" from a favorite *Seinfeld* episode. The rest of the class did *not* think I was funny and I pretty much forgot about the whole mantra thing until the night I went into labor. At some point during the middle of the night I found myself repeating the words "just one minute" during my contractions. It wasn't just the words that comforted me, but the reminder to keep myself present

ASK AN *expert*

Q: **What are some gentle prenatal yoga poses I can do?**

A: Doing yoga in the months leading up to and following labor can be beneficial for a number of reasons. Yoga helps improve flexibility and breathing capacity, reduces stress, builds strength, and enhances calm. Yoga techniques for mindfulness learned during pregnancy can also help through the pain of labor and postpartum anxiety. Prenatal yoga can include anything you feel comfortable doing, and if you already have an established practice, feel free to continue and modify as the teacher suggests. The following postures are perfect for beginners and seasoned practitioners alike, and take into account the needs of a pregnant woman's changing body. Always consult your doctor before engaging in new forms of physical activity, and stop if you don't feel well.

—Sara Kleinsmith, *certified yoga teacher,*
www.sarakleinsmith.com

Wall-Facing Dog

Downward dog is a beautiful, elemental pose of yoga, but pregnancy can cause some to feel dizzy when the head is down. This dog is a sensible alternative and providesmany of the benefits of downward dog, while also gently working the core. Place both hands on the wall at chest height. Walk the feet back and lean the hips away from the wall (stick your butt out). We're aiming to make an L shape with the body; think flat back, straight (ish) legs.

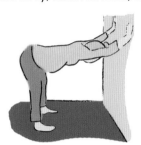

Breathe deeply. This is a lovely stretch for the back and hips, as well as shoulders and backs of the legs, and can be done easily on a lunch break or flight layover.

Wall Lunge

This posture is a gentle version of low lunge. It is designed to stretch the hip flexors and front of the body. Because the belly stretches in pregnancy, deep back bends may feel too intense. This is an accessible and effective alternative. Stand facing a wall and place both hands at chest height. Keep the left leg close to the wall and step the right leg back. Feet should be parallel, so that as you step the right foot back, the heel is off the floor. Deeply bend the left knee toward the wall and lift the chest to keep the upper body straight. Breathe deeply. At least

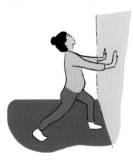

three long breaths are recommended, but stay for as long as you'd like. For a challenge, lift arms away from the wall, reaching them to the ceiling. Hold and breathe. Switch legs when finished.

Ankle Over Knee

This can be done seated on the floor or reclined. I prefer the chair variation for pregnancy, since being reclined is, at times, uncomfortable and not recommended. Sit tall at the front of your chair and take a deep breath. Remaining tall through the spine, cross your right ankle over your left knee. This is meant to stretch the external rotators of the hip, or outer hip, and may help to stave off sciatic nerve pain often associated with pregnancy. Gently lean forward with a "diagonal," not rounded, spine. Take several breaths. Make sure to leave space for the belly; you need not fold completely down to feel the stretch.

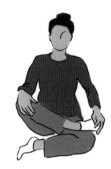

Seated Twist

This twist can be done sitting on the floor or in a chair. Spinal twists in pregnancy can be done, but care must be taken so that mommy and baby have space to move and breathe. This twist focuses on the upper trunk, thoracic spine, and shoulder blades. Sitting up tall in a chair or cross-legged on the floor, take a deep breath in. Lift both arms above your head and rotate the spine (twist) to face your right. The right hand comes to the back of the chair, and the left hand can rest on top of the right knee. Look over your right shoulder behind you. Working on "growing tall" and deeply breathing, hold this posture for several breaths.

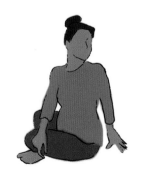
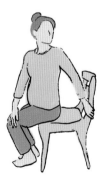

and focused on the moment at hand. My mantra helped keep me from feeling panicked or overwhelmed, and I'm grateful that I was able to come up with something so helpful to me—even if it was at the last minute!

Some other suggestions (that are probably more helpful than a *Seinfeld* quote) for birth mantras:

» I am strong. I am brave. I am okay.
» Open. Open. Open.
» Release.
» Down. Down. Down.
» I can do this.

It doesn't have to be especially brilliant or creative, but picking positive words to focus on can be a good alternative to other things you might be thinking like "This hurts" or "I can't do this." If you are religious, finding a short and simple prayer or verse can be a great choice too. Do you have a favorite quote that makes you feel calm and confident? Books, songs, favorite movies, or historical figures can be great sources of inspiration. Most mamas find short and simple mantras to be the most helpful.

SETTING GOALS

Even before baby actually arrives, parenthood is all about goals. Some of the best advice I remember getting as an expectant mother was to spend my time focusing on what kind of parent I'd like to be rather than dreaming about what kind of child I'd like to have. I took this to heart, and spent countless hours thinking about how I would care for and raise my child.

My goals were incredibly idealistic, and the reality of being a mom brought many of my loftiest ambitions down closer to earth. For example, before my son was born I read everything I could on a practice called elimination communication. Inspired by seeing the practice in action while living abroad, I was determined to have him potty trained from birth. As of this writing, he is now 3 years old and flat-out refuses to toilet train. So you see, we can't win them all!

Even if you can't reach every goal you set as a new parent, I think it's healthy to have an ideal to reach toward. Just don't be too hard on yourself if it doesn't work out exactly the way you pictured. For every goal that falls short, another will succeed, and every attempt was surely worth the effort.

GETTING POSTPARTUM SUPPORT

No matter who you are, what your delivery was like, how healthy your baby is, or what your life is like, there is one universal truth among mothers. Having a baby is very, very hard work. It's true for all of us, and each in our own completely unique way. The challenges that you face during your postpartum period may be completely different than those of your best friend, mother, or sister.

The first three months of a child's life can be extremely challenging. Not only is your body recovering physically, you may find yourself processing a huge amount of raw emotion as you bond with baby and navigate life with a whole new set of rules. And all of this while suffering from a lack of sleep and going through some pretty intense hormonal changes!

During the postpartum period, support is key. Before your baby arrives, spend some time thinking about what kind of support is available to you and start making plans and arrangements to make sure that support is there when you need it. What kind of help should you ask for? You're likely to need help with everything from laundry and cooking to babysitting and emotional support. Here are a few thoughts on where you can get support:

Your Spouse or Partner: Every family is different, so having a spouse or partner to lean on after baby's arrival isn't possible for every mama. If your spouse or partner is present during the postpartum period they are likely to be your number one source of daily support. Make sure to take some time before the birth to discuss how you both plan to approach the workload of caring for mama and baby. Be clear about your needs and expectations. Remember that this is a life-changing experience for both of you and you'll need to be caring and patient with one another as you go through this journey side by side. Communication, both before and after baby arrives, is key!

Family and Friends: If you are lucky enough to have family who is willing to help with baby, be sure to take full advantage. Make sure your family knows exactly what kind of help you expect, when and where that help is needed, and from whom. Make your expectations and boundaries clear and have these conversations well before baby's arrival.

ESSENTIAL OILS COMMONLY USED DURING PREGNANCY[1]

SCIENTIFIC (INCI) NAME	PROPERTIES	USAGE RATE (Less than 1% in any application / 4 drops or less per bath)
Chamomile, Roman	*Chamaemelum nobile*	Anti-inflammatory, calming, soothing
Geranium	*Pelargonium graveolens*	Balancing
Lavender	*Lavandula angustifolia*	Anti-bacterial
Rose Otto	*Rosa centifolia*	Balancing
Sandalwood	*Santalum album*	Calming, soothing
Sweet Orange	*Citrus sinensis*	Anti-bacterial, astringent, uplifting
Tea Tree	*Melaleuca alternifolia*	Anti-bacterial
Ylang Ylang	*Cananga odorata*	Balancing, uplifting

Often family members want to help, but without clear instructions they may not know how!

Social Circle: Make a habit of calling or texting your closest friends and family and ask them to also check in with you during the first months with baby. Women can sometimes feel isolated during the postpartum period, so simply having someone to talk to can be immensely helpful.

Postpartum Doulas, Night Nurses, and Mother's Helpers: If family isn't available and if finances allow, you may want to consider hiring help for the first few days, weeks, or months. Choose a reputable service with plenty of solid credentials and make whatever arrangements you can ahead of time. You can schedule interviews, book service, and do research all before your baby is born. If you find yourself feeling overwhelmed after baby arrives you will know exactly who to call.

Meal Trains or Care Calendars: There are quite a few Web sites that allow your family and friends to coordinate easily to provide meals, babysitting, and household help after baby arrives. If possible, get a friend to set this up for you and communicate with contributors on your behalf.

Your OBGYN or Midwife: It's a good idea to keep in touch with your healthcare providers so that they can check on your physical and mental well-being. If you begin feeling overwhelmed or depressed,

these are people who can help get you the care and resources you need to make things better.

Support Groups: Before baby arrives, look up support groups for breast-feeding or new mothers in your area and write down their meeting dates, times, and locations. Sometimes the best way to get through the postpartum period is by connecting with other women who are going through the same thing.

HOW TO ADD ESSENTIAL OILS TO BATH & BODY RECIPES

I chose not to add essential oils to the bath and body recipes in this book for one very important reason: There is no guarantee that any essential oil is always safe for all women in all pregnancies. While there are plenty of essential oils (the most popular of which I have listed in the chart here) that are commonly used during pregnancy without incident, it's important to remember that these are highly potent substances with powerful properties and the results aren't always predictable. To learn more about essential oil safety, visit The National Association for Holistic Aromatherapy's Web site at naha.org.

If you have any health conditions, whether they are related to your pregnancy or not, I urge you to consult your doctor or midwife before using any essential oils, even those listed here. If you do decide to add essential oils to the skin or hair care recipes in this chapter, be sure to follow the usage rates indicated. You know what they say about too much of a good thing, right?

ABOUT STRETCH MARKS

Well, mama, I'm sorry to tell you this, but you just might get stretch marks. Even with the very best belly butter applied systematically, there's just no way to guarantee an unmarred belly by the time baby arrives. According to doctors, genetics play a huge part in a woman's tendency to see stretch marks.

Another very big and totally unpredictable factor is how baby will grow, and how the womb will be positioned in your body. Some women never develop stretch marks, while others see them with every pregnancy. It's even possible to skip stretch marks during one pregnancy then be bombarded during the next! I made it all the way to thirty-eight weeks before seeing a mark, then woke up one morning with tiger stripes across my pelvis.

This might seem a little scary, but if you do end up developing stretch marks, I challenge you to see them as beauty marks instead of scars. Your body goes through an amazing transformation when it makes a child, and the marks left behind are proof of just how incredible you really are. In the meantime, try to focus on keeping your skin healthy by moisturizing it at least twice a day and keeping your body nourished and hydrated by eating well and drinking plenty of water. Take good care of that marvelous body of yours, tiger stripes and all.

---

handmade mama tip

HER EXPERIENCE IS NOT YOUR EXPERIENCE

While you are preparing for baby, you are likely to be surrounded by a chorus of very different (and often contradictory) voices. Motherhood is pretty intense. For a lot of women, it is one of the most defining and life-changing experiences of their lives. When something that huge happens, it can't help but come along with an enormous pile of feelings—feelings that are just dying to come out and be shared with others.

Mamas will want to share their stories with you—to open up and spill out their hard-earned wisdom and well-intentioned warnings or predictions. You'll hear birth stories that inspire you, and others that scare you. Parents will shower you with their best tips, secret weapons, and trusted techniques for dealing with everything from sleepless nights to stubborn toddlers. Some people will delight in reminding you that you are in for a challenge while others will paint you a picture so perfect that it's almost guaranteed to disappoint.

No matter what anyone tells you, remember this—your experience is not her experience. When you hear words like "always" or "never," stick an asterisk next to the sentence. Every mama is an expert on her *own* baby. Every birth story is special. Yours will be too.

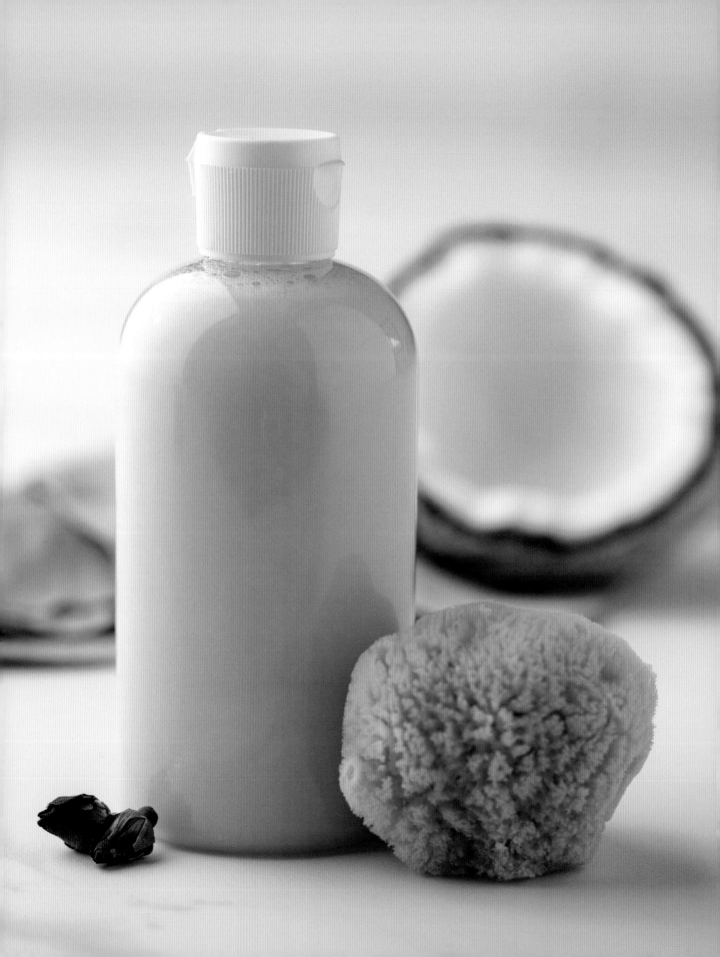

HEAD TO TOE MAMA WASH

YIELD: *About 1½ cups (355 ml)*

Are the parabens in your shampoo starting to freak you out? Are the synthetic fragrances in your body wash making you cringe every time you hop in the shower? These kinds of ingredients have been related to some pretty scary stuff, like allergies, hormone disruption, and even cancer.

But fear not, beautiful mama—this all-in-one liquid soap recipe has got you covered. With a rich lather, a gentle touch, and a neutral aroma, you can give your shampoo, body wash, and even shaving cream the boot. The best part? This simple formula is completely free of sketchy synthetic ingredients.

INGREDIENTS

- 1 cup (240 ml) liquid castile soap
- ½ cup (120 ml) canned unsweetened coconut milk
- 1 tablespoon (15 ml) Herbal Body Oil (recipe on page 26)

DIRECTIONS

1. Combine ingredients in a 12-ounce squirt bottle and shake well.
2. Store at room temperature for up to 1 week, or refrigerate for up to 3 months.

TO USE

Squirt the mixture liberally onto a washcloth or shower pouf to use as body wash. To use as shampoo, apply up to one tablespoon of the mixture to your hair. Lather, rinse with water, then follow with Apple Cider Vinegar Rinse (page 45) to remove excess residue. To use as shaving cream, simply work up a rich lather of soap between your hands then smooth over slightly moistened skin.

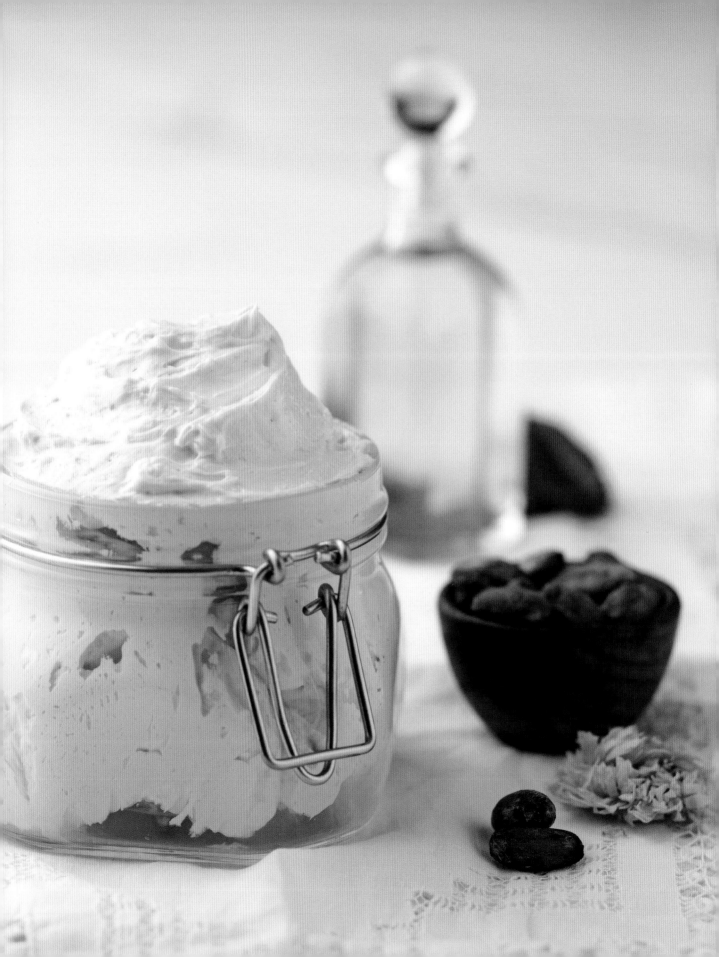

WHIPPED BELLY BUTTER

YIELD: *About 1 cup (240 ml)*

As a pregnant mama, one of the most extraordinary things you will witness is the awe-inspiring transformation of your body. As baby grows, so does your belly. At times it can seem that weeks have gone by without a visible change. Other times a baby bump seems to grow overnight—or right before your eyes!

All of this magical expansion asks a lot from our skin. Keeping your belly well-moisturized with high-quality whole ingredients is a great way to offer your body support during this incredible process. As your skin stretches to accommodate baby, it can feel itchy, irritated, and sometimes even a little painful. This kind of discomfort often indicates that the belly needs a little extra love.

As a rule, it's best to apply belly butter at least twice every day, and again any time you feel itchy or uncomfortable. As you get into your third trimester, make sure to moisturize not only your tummy, but also your pelvis, bikini area, breasts, and hips—all of which may be experiencing big changes as baby's arrival approaches.

If you prefer a scented belly butter, try incorporating the Herbal Body Oil on page 26. If you'd prefer to keep things simple, plain apricot kernel oil will do just fine.

INGREDIENTS

- ½ cup (120 ml) shea,* cupuacu, or mango butter (room temperature)
- 2 ounces (60 ml) apricot kernel oil or Herbal Body Oil (recipe on page 26)
- 1 ounce (30 ml) avocado oil
- 1 ounce (30 ml) argan oil

*Shea butter shares a common chemical with the proteins in natural latex. If you are at all sensitive to latex, I'd recommend making this recipe with another type of vegetable butter. My favorites are semi-soft butters like cupuacu or mango butter.

DIRECTIONS

1. Place the butter in the bowl of a stand mixer fitted with the whisk attachment.

2. Whisk the butter on medium speed for about 5 minutes. The butter should become soft and fluffy.

3. Stop the mixer, add the oils, and whisk on low speed for about 30 seconds. The oils should be thoroughly mixed into the butter.

4. Stop the mixer, scrape down the sides of the bowl, and then bring the mixer up to high speed. Whip the butter for 5 to 10 minutes, until it becomes thicker, light in color, and very fluffy. The butter should form stiff peaks, like buttercream frosting, when it is finished.

5. Spoon the butter into a jar. The mixture will become slightly firmer as it cools and sets over the next few hours, but will remain relatively soft and fluffy. During hot weather, the butter may soften and lose its fluffy texture. Try keeping it an air-conditioned room or in the fridge to protect it.

TO USE

Apply belly butter liberally to your stomach, pelvis, bikini area, breasts, and hips twice a day, or as often as needed (anytime your belly feels tight or itchy). Massage the butter into your skin in a gentle, circular motion. The butter will take a little extra time to absorb compared with commercial lotion, so be sure to give the conditioning oils and butters enough time to soak in before getting dressed.

APPLE CIDER VINEGAR RINSE

YIELD: *About 1 cup (240 ml)*

Following a natural shampoo like the Head to Toe Mama Wash (page 40) with this Apple Cider Vinegar Rinse is essential to the success of your natural hair care routine. The rinse will help to remove any leftover soap residue, balance your scalp's pH, and reduce tangles—leaving your hair soft, silky, and happy as can be.

INGREDIENTS

» 1 tablespoon (15 ml) apple cider vinegar

» 1 cup (240 ml) water

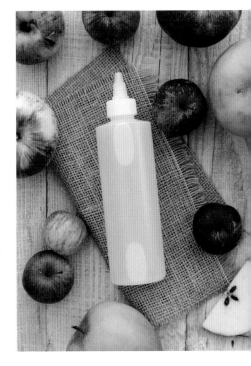

DIRECTIONS

1. Combine ingredients in an 8-ounce squirt bottle and shake well.

2. Store at room temperature for up to 1 week, or refrigerate for up to 3 months.

HOW TO USE

After washing and rinsing your hair, douse it liberally with vinegar rinse. Massage the rinse into your hair, then let it sit for at least a minute. I like to leave the rinse on as I wash up, then rinse it before leaving the shower. When you rinse, make sure to do so very well. A thorough rinse will keep your hair from smelling like vinegar when it dries.

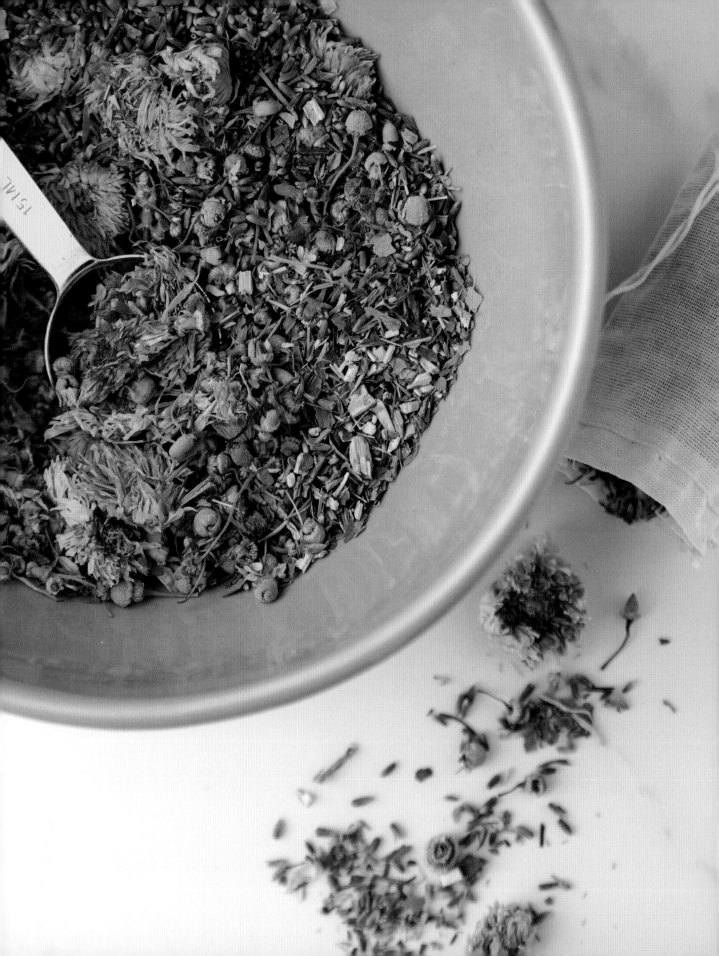

POSTPARTUM HERB BATH

YIELD: *2 quarts (1.89 L)*

There are a few gnarly parts of childbirth that are hard to ever really be prepared for. For me, the gnarliest part of all was what midwives like to call "The Ring of Fire." That's when the baby's head starts to poke its way out of your lady parts. It hurts. A lot.

For some mamas, this painful part of childbirth also acts as a motivator. This is the time when some mothers get to reach down and feel the fuzz of their baby's hair for the very first time. If you aren't too squeamish you may even get to take a peek using a small mirror. Knowing your baby is right there often helps mothers make it through that final exhausting push.

Though you and your doctor or midwife will surely do everything possible to keep your precious perineum (that's the thin strip of skin between your anus and vagina) intact as baby's head pushes through, you won't always succeed. Frankly, tears and episiotomies are a very typical part of childbirth, and while it may be excruciating at the time, the body will and does heal after it's over.

Whether or not you need stitches after birth, your vagina and perineum will have gone through a lot by the time you get home. While you won't be able to soak in a clawfoot tub anytime soon, you can dip your most delicate parts in a sitz bath of soothing herbs and salts to help soothe pain and encourage healing. This mixture is also an incredible replacement for plain water in perineum bottles used to cleanse stitches.

INGREDIENTS

- 2 quarts (1.89 L) water
- ¼ cup (60 g) sea salt
- ¼ cup (8 g) dried lavender buds
- ½ cup (15 g) dried chamomile
- ½ cup (30 g) dried calendula
- ½ cup (30 g) dried plantain leaf

POSTPARTUM HERB BATH *(continued)*

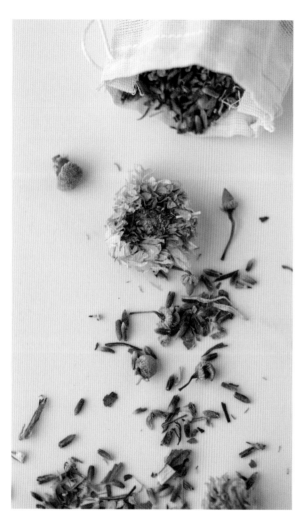

DIRECTIONS

1. Bring water to a boil in large pot, then turn off heat to stop boiling.

2. Add salt and herbs and allow to steep until cool (about 30 minutes).

3. Strain and discard herbs.

4. Store infused water in a ½-gallon (2 L) pitcher and refrigerate between uses.

TO USE

There are several different ways to make use of this soothing herbal infusion.

- Fill your peri-bottle with a mixture of 1 part herb bath and 1 part hot sterile water, then use as directed by caregiver.
- Fill a sitz bath with 1 part herb bath and 1 part hot sterile water, then soak until the water cools (about 15 minutes) once per day.
- Soak sani-pads with herb bath before putting them into the freezer. The cold pads can be used like ice packs on sore lady parts.

BUCKWHEAT SLEEP MASK

YIELD: *1 sleep mask*

Sleep when your baby sleeps: This is easily one of the most repeated bits of advice that new mothers will hear during the first few months of their child's life. While it is a good strategy since you certainly won't be sleeping while the baby is awake, it's also one of those things that is a whole lot easier said than done.

First off, there are a few other things you might want to do while baby is sleeping, like eat, shower, or spend a few precious minutes in solitude. When you do want to take a nap, it can sometimes be difficult to wind down or drift off, as most of us are not used to sleeping during the day or amidst the noise of a busy household. A sleep mask can help. The dampened light and gentle pressure of buckwheat hulls will provide you with a bit of tranquility—hopefully enough to aid in a quick and easy journey to dreamland.

MATERIALS + TOOLS

- ⅓ yard (30.5cm) flannel
- ⅓ yard (30.5cm) cotton batting
- 18 in. (45cm) length of ½-in. (1.25mm) elastic
- About ½ cup (120 ml) or ½ ounce (15 g) buckwheat hulls
- Matching thread
- Tracing paper and pencil
- Scissors or a rotary cutter with mat
- Pins
- Ruler or measuring tape
- Sewing machine
- Hand sewing needle

DIRECTIONS

Measure and Cut Pattern Pieces

1. Cut or trace pattern pieces (Eye Pillow A, Eye Pillow B) from pattern library (page 192).

2. Fold flannel in half. Pin pattern piece Eye Pillow A to fabric, with arrow against fold. Cut fabric. Repeat to make two matching pieces.

3. Fold batting in half. Pin pattern piece Eye Pillow B to batting, with arrow against fold. Cut batting, and repeat to make two matching pieces.

4. Measure and cut one 1½ x 24-inch (4 x 61cm) piece of flannel. This will be the strap.

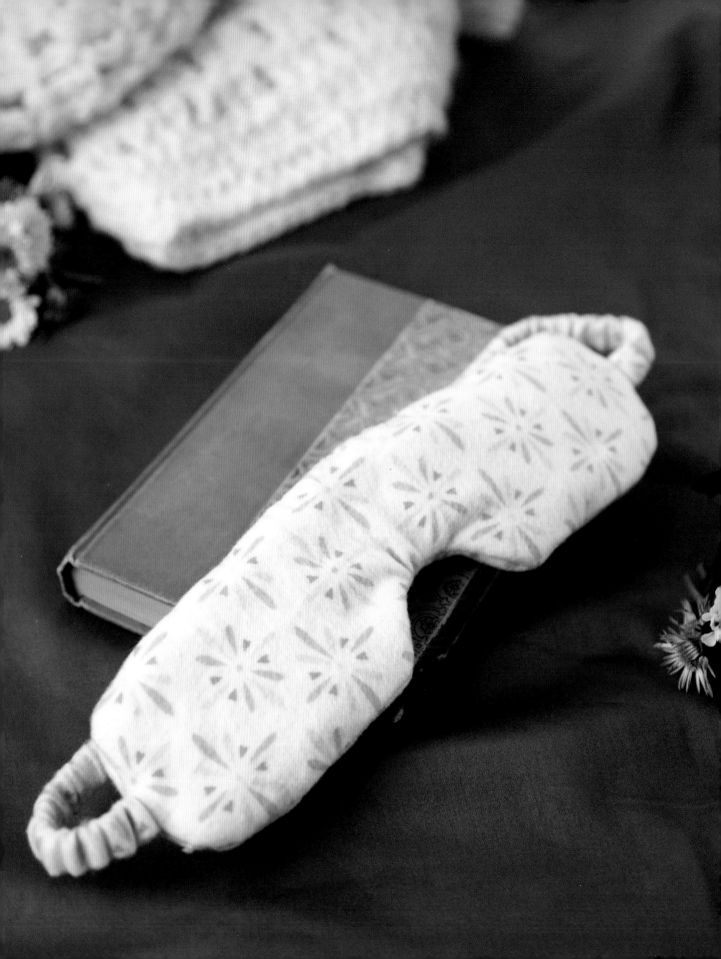

BUCKWHEAT SLEEP MASK *(continued)*

Make Strap

5. With right sides in, fold strap in half lengthwise and pin. Stitch up the side, leaving the top and bottom open for turning (see figure 1, page 52).

6. Turn out strap (instructions on page 20). Thread elastic through strap, pinning one end of elastic to each end of strap. Fabric will be bunched in between.

Assemble Pillow

7. Pin cut batting to the wrong side of cut flannel. Stitch around edges of batting, securing batting to wrong side of flannel. Repeat with second piece (see figure 2, page 52).

8. Place right sides of eye pillow together. Place one end of strap in between pillow pieces with short end sticking out. Pin to secure strap, then stitch that side closed (see figure 3, page 52).

9. Check sizing on elastic band to make sure it will fit comfortably on your head. Snip off an inch or two as needed.

10. Pin the other strap into the mask with the raw edge of the strap poking out. Pin around the edges of the mask and stitch all the way around, leaving a 2-inch (5cm) opening for turning out. Be careful not to sew over the strap inside the mask (see figure 4, page 52).

Finish Sleep Mask

11. Turn out sleep mask and fill with buckwheat hulls.

12. Hand-stitch the opening shut (instructions on page 19).

TO USE

Place the sleep mask over your eyes before nap time or bed time. Mask may be chilled in the freezer or heated for 30 seconds in the microwave to help soothe headaches or tired eyes.

BUCKWHEAT SLEEP MASK (continued)

Figure 1

Figure 2

Figure 3

Figure 4

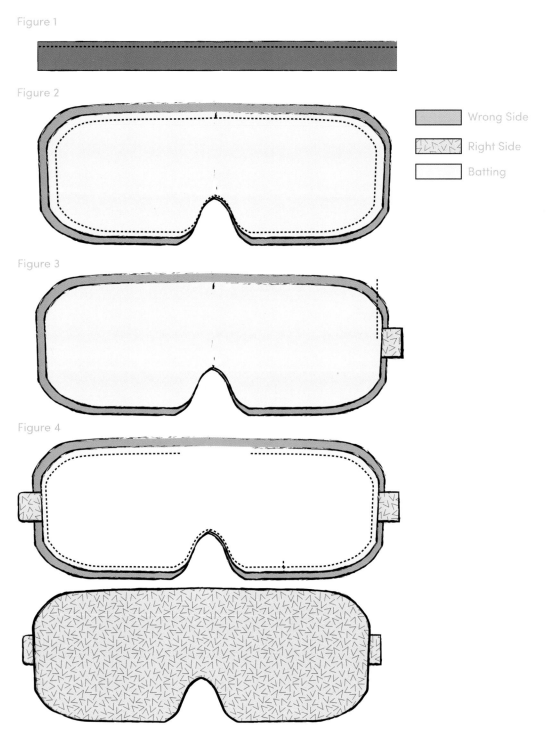

Wrong Side

Right Side

Batting

BUCKWHEAT PILLOWS

YIELD: *1 buckwheat pillow*

t's no secret that neither pregnancy nor childbirth are pain-free ventures. Each part of the motherhood journey comes with its fair share of aches and pains. Thankfully, soothing a sore muscle is a whole lot more straight-forward than soothing a cranky child!

Ice, heat, massage, and rest is often all that's needed to fix things up. Buckwheat pillows are light and flexible, making them perfect for soothing stiff muscles. They can be heated gently to provide a warm compress, or chilled in the freezer to serve as an ice pack.

Buckwheat pillows are also helpful for baby care. Gentle heat can often help babies release gas and relax tied-up tummies. Just be sure to use very mild heat when caring for little ones.

MATERIALS + TOOLS

- ¼ yard (23cm) flannel
- ¼ yard (23cm) cotton batting
- About 2 cups (475 ml) / 5 ounces (150g) buckwheat hulls
- Matching thread
- Tracing paper and pencil
- Scissors or a rotary cutter with mat
- Pins
- Sewing machine
- Hand sewing needle

DIRECTIONS

Cut Pattern Pieces

1. Cut or trace pattern pieces (Buckwheat Pillow A) from pattern library (page 191).

2. Fold flannel in half. Pin pattern piece Buckwheat Pillow to fabric, with arrow against fold. Cut fabric, and repeat to make two matching pieces.

3. Fold batting in half. Pin the same pattern piece to batting, with arrow against fold. Cut batting, and repeat to make two matching pieces.

Assemble Pillow

4. Place right sides of flannel together, and a layer of batting above and below the flannel. The order should be batting, flannel, flannel, batting.

5. Pin edges and sew all four layers together around edges, leaving a 2-inch (5cm) opening to turn out pillow (see figure 1, page 54).

BUCKWHEAT PILLOWS *(continued)*

Finish Pillow

6. Turn out pillow (instructions on page 20) and fill with buckwheat hulls.

7. Hand-stitch opening closed (instructions on page 19).

TO USE

Warm pillow in microwave for 30 seconds or chill in freezer for at least 1 hour. Test for safety of temperature before application.

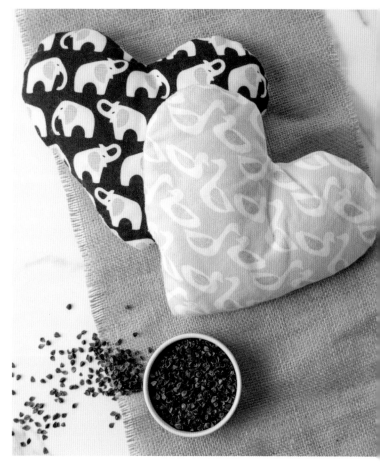

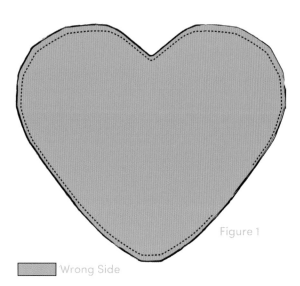

Figure 1

Wrong Side

NURSING PADS

YIELD: *12 nursing pads (6 pairs)*

Let's not mince words. Some of us are gushers—our bosoms exploding with milk upon the mere thought of our babies. While having an abundance of milk is a blessing in many ways, it can also be a hassle. And at times, it can be downright embarrassing. To help keep blouses dry and bedsheets clean, some of us need a little extra help.

Nursing pads act as a barrier and can help maintain a clean and dry environment, discouraging bacteria that can lead to uncomfortable complications like blocked ducts or mastitis. Keeping a small stockpile on hand allows you to replace soaked pads as needed. On an extra-milky day, some mamas can go through as many as ten pairs of pads! Even after your milk production has started to calm down, the occasional leak can still happen, so many mamas choose to continue wearing breast pads as long as they are actively nursing little ones.

You have the option of either using a top stitch or a zigzag stitch when finishing these. The top stitch is the easier choice, as this is the most commonly used stitch, and familiar to even beginner sewers. If you are up for something new, try using a tight zigzag stitch to finish the edges. This will help reduce fraying and give the pads a longer life.

I used a combination of flannel and bamboo fleece to make my nursing pads. If you prefer, the bamboo fleece can be swapped for cotton flannel or terrycloth. If you'd like your pads to be extra water resistant, try using PUL fabric (the same material used to make diaper covers) in place of flannel.

MATERIALS + TOOLS

- ¼ yard (23cm) flannel
- ¼ yard (23cm) bamboo fleece
- ¼ yard (23cm) cotton batting
- Matching thread
- Tracing paper and pencil
- Scissors or a rotary cutter with mat
- Pins
- Sewing machine

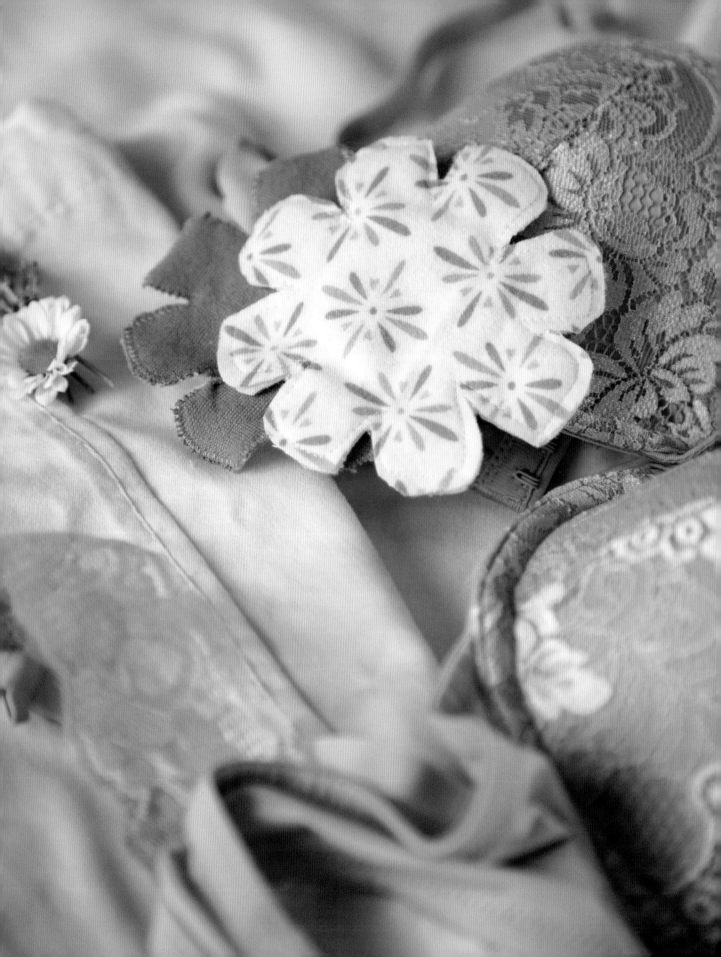

NURSING PADS *(continued)*

DIRECTIONS

Cut Pattern Pieces

1. Cut or trace pattern pieces (Breast Pads A, Breast Pads B) from pattern library (page 189).

2. Pin pattern piece Nursing Pad A to fabric. Cut fabric. Repeat to make eleven more pieces.

3. Pin pattern piece Nursing Pad B to cotton batting. Cut batting. Repeat to make eleven more pieces.

Assemble Pad

4. Match up two pieces of flannel with wrong sides together, and right side facing out. Place one circle of batting between the two layers, in the center of the pad. Pin edges.

Finish Pad

5. Stitch around edges using either a top stitch or narrow zigzag stitch. Use a ⅛-inch (3mm) seam allowance, sewing as close to the edge as possible.

6. Trim any excess fabric from edges.

Finish Batch

7. Repeat steps 4 through 6 to make eleven more pads.

TO USE

Place nursing pad over nipple under bra or sleep bra. Replace when wet. Pads should be washed in warm or cold water with gentle detergent and dried on low heat.

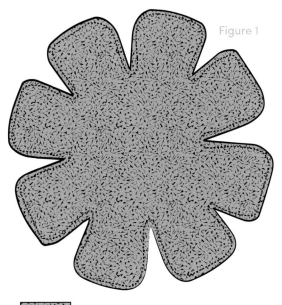

Figure 1

Right Side

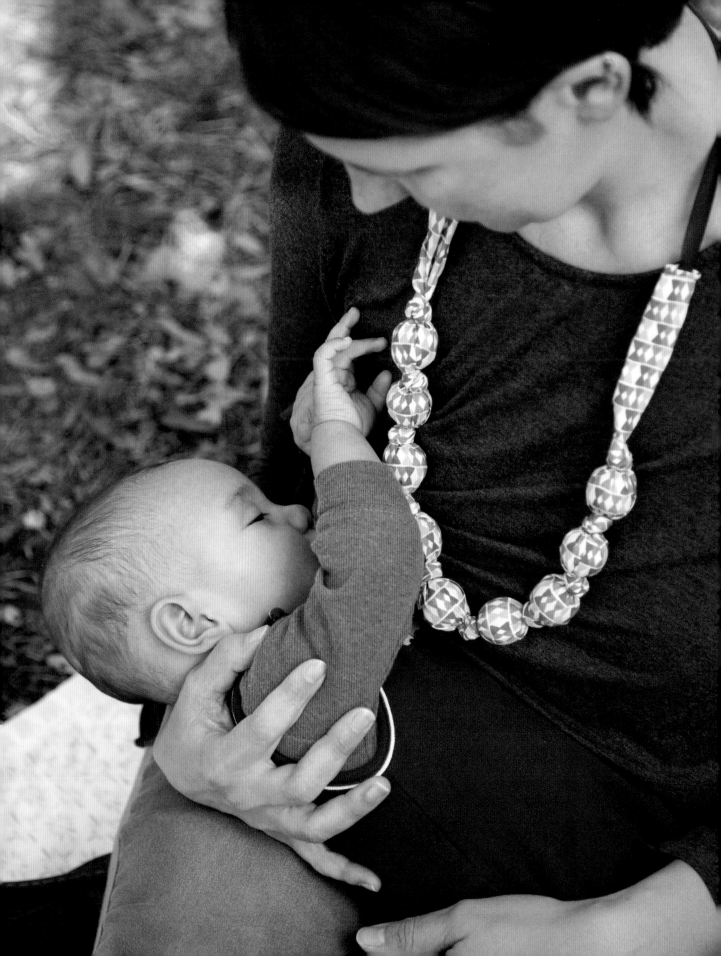

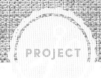

NURSING NECKLACE

YIELD: *1 nursing necklace*

If you've ever been nipped by puppy teeth you know how sharp tiny things can be. A baby's fingernails, for example, can cause a shocking amount of pain—especially when dug into the tender flesh of mama's booby! Little babies quickly become adept at torturing their mothers when it's time to nurse. The more aware of the world they become, the more ways they discover to make breast-feeding a challenge.

When my sweet little bundle first fish-hooked my nostril, I knew it was time for a change. While I was determined to keep breast-feeding, I was also really tired of being pinched, poked, and scratched during every feeding. I was exceedingly grateful when my sister lent me her nursing necklace.

Nursing necklaces are a great way to distract babies while they eat. The bumpy texture of fabric and wooden beads give baby something to grab—something highly preferable to poor mom. This simple necklace will also come in handy when baby starts teething. Little ones can happily gnaw this special necklace whenever they are feeling bitey.

MATERIALS + TOOLS

- 2 10-in. (25cm) pieces of ¼-in. (6mm)-wide satin ribbon
- 9 large wooden beads
- ⅛ yard (11.5mm) calico or quilter's cotton
- Matching thread
- Pins
- Ruler or measuring tape
- Scissors
- Sewing machine

DIRECTIONS

Measure and Cut Pattern Pieces

1. Measure and cut one 4 x 44-inch (10 x 111cm) strip of fabric.

Create Tube

2. Fold fabric in half (lengthwise) with right sides together.

3. Pin fabric and stitch up the long side, leaving ends open for turning.

4. Turn out fabric (instructions on page 20).

NURSING NECKLACE *(continued)*

Attach Ribbon

5. Tuck in about 1 inch (2.5cm) of fabric on one side of the tube, and slip the end of one piece of ribbon into the tucked side. Fold the tucked side in half and pin it to secure.

6. Stitch the tucked, folded side shut (see figure 1, below).

Add Beads

7. Tie a knot in the tube of fabric about 3 inches (7.5cm) from the stitched end.

8. Place a wooden bead inside the tube and push it down until it reaches the knot. Tie a second knot directly after the bead, keeping the knots and beads as close together as you can.

9. Repeat with the eight remaining beads.

Attach Ribbon

10. Tuck in about 1 inch (2.5cm) of fabric at the end of the tube and slip the end of one piece of ribbon inside. Fold the tucked side in half, and pin it to secure.

11. Stitch the tucked, folded side shut (see figure 2, below).

TO USE

Tie ribbons together to secure necklace. Wear necklace during nursing sessions, when carrying a feisty baby, or any time you please.

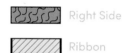 Right Side

Ribbon

Figure 1

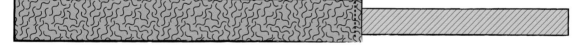

Figure 2

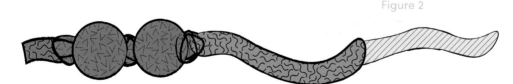

MOON PADS

YIELD: *6 moon pads*

After enjoying forty weeks of freedom from one's monthly curse, it seems a bit unfair to be saddled with weeks of bleeding after childbirth. Alas, such is life, and by this time every mother knows that womanhood is not without its discomforts.

Reusable cloth pads can help to make the experience a little more comfortable, and have the added virtue of reducing plastic waste. For mamas with sensitive skin (like myself), these soft flannel pads are a real treasure.

This pattern uses two layers of batting for general use, but you can easily customize the pads to suit your own needs and preferences by reducing or increasing the number of batting inserts used. For a heavy flow, try using four inserts. For a very light flow, try using just one. If you want to reinforce your pads with a waterproof layer, try lining the bottoms with PUL fabric.

MATERIALS + TOOLS

- ¼ yard (23cm) flannel
- ¼ yard (23cm) cotton batting
- 6 metal snaps
- Matching thread
- Tracing paper and pencil
- Scissors or a rotary cutter with mat
- Pins
- Ruler or measuring tape
- Sewing machine
- Hand sewing needle

DIRECTIONS

Measure and Cut Pattern Pieces

1. Cut or trace pattern pieces (Moon Pad A, Moon Pad B) from pattern library (page 189).

2. Fold flannel in half. Pin pattern piece Moon Pad A to fabric, with arrow against fold. Cut fabric. Repeat to make two matching pieces.

3. Fold batting in half. Pin pattern piece Moon Pad B to batting, with arrow against fold. Cut batting. Repeat to make two matching pieces.

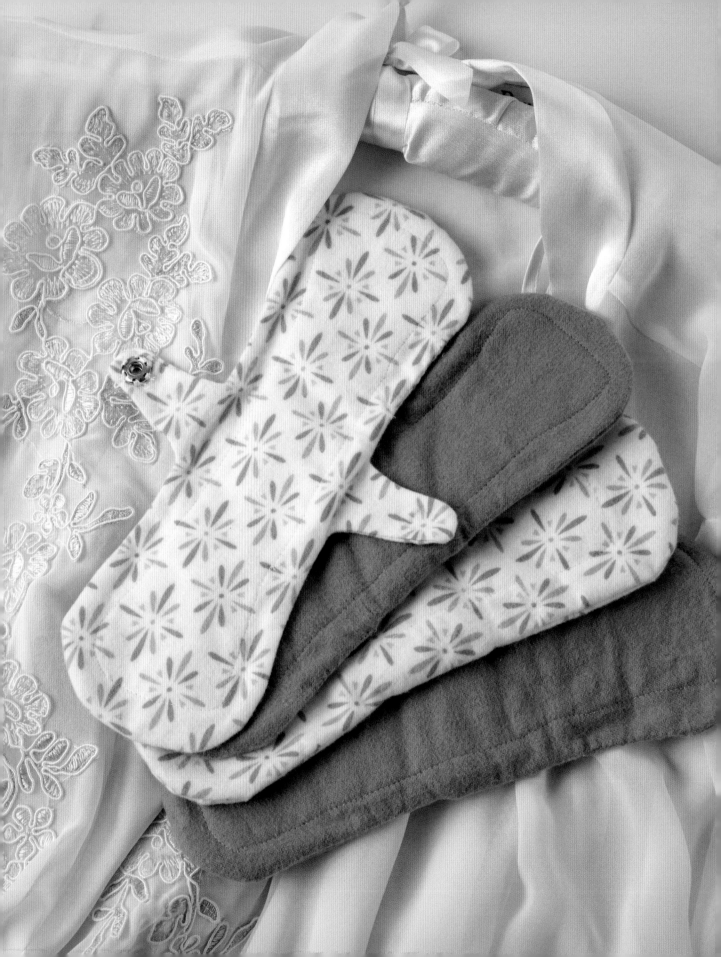

MOON PADS *(continued)*

Assemble Pad

4. Pin cut batting to the wrong side of cut flannel. Stitch around edges of batting, securing batting to wrong side of flannel. Repeat with second piece (see figure 1, below).

5. Place right sides of the moon pad together. Stitch all the way around, leaving a 2-inch (5cm) opening for turning out (see figure 2, below).

Finish Pad

6. Turn out the moon pad and hand-stitch the opening shut (instructions on pages 19–20).

7. Hand-stitch metal snaps onto wings.

Finish Batch

8. Repeat to make five more pads.

TO USE

Place in underwear as you would a disposable maxi pad and snap in place. Rinse moon pads with water immediately after use, and wash in bulk with hot water and detergent. Dry on low or medium heat.

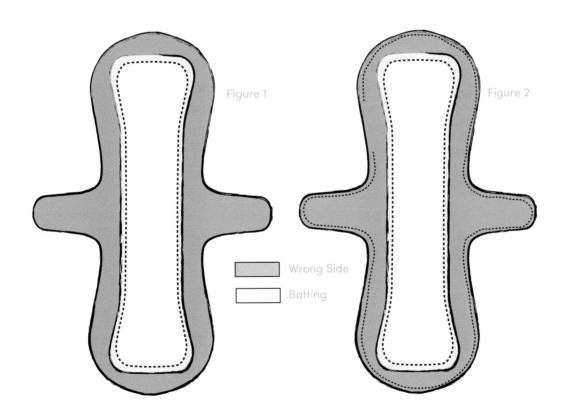

Figure 1

Figure 2

Wrong Side

Batting

PERSONAL STORY

Charlie's birth story

Like so many parts of my motherhood journey, the birth of my son, Charlie, didn't go exactly as expected. My labor started around sunset on May 26 and by 10 a.m. on May 27, I was holding a tiny (extra tiny—only 5 pounds and 6 ounces) baby in my arms. No one expected him to come so quickly—not myself and certainly not my doula or midwife.

In fact, nobody realized how close I was to giving birth as I calmly waddled into the birth center where Charlie was born. It wasn't until the midwife took a look down below that she realized what was happening. Women who are about to push, I was informed, don't usually arrive cracking jokes or waiting patiently to be told what happens next.

I was also told for months before Charlie was born that my contractions would come in regular intervals well before active labor began. The reason that I only arrived at the birth center minutes before starting to push was that I had been waiting for my contractions to come five minutes apart. That never happened for me, and so I ended up spending the night laboring alone in my bathroom, foot propped up on the tub, breathing through contractions and waiting for *real* labor to start.

It wasn't until I hit transition that I decided to stop taking no for an answer, and that it was time to go to the birth center whether my midwife thought I was ready or not. It had rained hard in Austin the night before, and roads were closed all across the city. As a result, my doula and the midwife delivering Charlie were delayed. When we finally arrived at the birth center, there was no one to let us in! I ended up laboring in the parking lot, leaning against my car, blearily observing the morning traffic as it whizzed by.

When they finally let us inside, I remember bracing myself, thinking that I still had to make it through active labor. I had no idea that the whole thing would be over and done with in just a couple of hours. When I lay down on the bed, I felt the first urge to push and my midwife looked up at me in utter surprise. "You are having this baby *now*," she said, and asked if I was ready to start pushing.

I figured that I was as ready as I was going to get, so agreed to let her break my waters and get started. A gush of warm liquid pre-empted an unstoppable urge to bear down and push. And push I did, propped up by my husband behind and my doula below; I pushed and pushed for around ninety minutes. My midwife did her best to keep me from tearing my perineum, but when it came time for me to push slowly I just couldn't control the urge. My muscles took on a mind of their own as my baby (who is just as intent on his goals today) made his way to the great wide world.

Charlie and I even finished the delivery with a surprise. As my birth team cheered me on, letting me know that we were just a handful of pushes away from the finish line, Charlie shot out all at once into the arms of my amazed midwife.

He was tiny—less than five and a half pounds, but fully developed and nearly a week overdue. When I delivered my placenta, it was similarly small—the smallest, the staff remarked, that they had ever seen. More than a year later I would have this little mystery explained by being diagnosed with a blood disorder called Factor V Leiden, and realize just how determined this little soul had been to get here. At the time, I simply basked in the wonder of my beautiful little child.

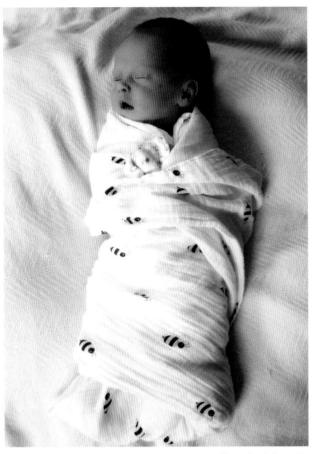

Photo: Sarah Kamalsky

Our family has had its share of challenges and heartaches since that morning in 2014, but no matter how hard it has been at times, I can honestly say these have been the best years of my life. Mama loves you, Charlie.

food & nutrition for mama

While it is important to have a good set of bath and body products to keep yourself feeling comfortable, during pregnancy it is also vital to nourish yourself with proper nutrition and healthy foods.

HYDRATION TIPS

One guarantee about this next section—by the time you finish reading it, you'll feel like I talk about drinking water a little too much. The amount of recipes included to increase hydration might seem a bit over the top, but drinking plenty of water really is one of the simplest ways to keep yourself feeling happy and healthy during pregnancy and through your postpartum period. Dehydration (even mild dehydration) can lead to headaches, pulled muscles, sore joints, clogged ducts, and fatigue. Your job of making and caring for another human being is hard enough without all of that. Still, drinking all that water can get old quick. Here are a few ways to help keep you on your game:

Treat Yourself to a Really Great Water Bottle: Whether you prefer a quart-sized mason jar or the latest and greatest athletic sports bottle, having a sturdy, portable water bottle that you are genuinely fond of will help a lot. And make sure that it holds enough water to keep you going while you work, run errands, or travel. Bonus points if the vessel fits in your car's cup holder!

There's an App for That: Actually, there are several, and plenty of them are free. Do a search on your phone for apps that are designed to help keep you motivated and hydrated with notifications, badges, and more.

Mix Things Up: Diminish hydration fatigue by drinking your water different ways. Try it with or without ice, hot or room temperature, flavored, infused, sparkling, frozen . . . You get the idea!

ASK AN *expert*

Q: **What are your favorite healthy alternatives for battling sugar and junk food cravings?**

A: Cravings are a real thing! My number one tip is to drink a full glass of water before reaching for anything. Oftentimes our bodies are dehydrated, and we hear the signal as hunger. If you still have the craving, opt for a high-quality decadent dark chocolate (70% cacao or higher). One square of this rich chocolate will curb your craving. Low-glycemic berries are a great option too: blueberries, raspberries, and strawberries. They go great paired with your dark chocolate too! Eating in moderation every single day will help with sugar cravings. The less of it you eat, the less your brain tells you that you "need" it.

—*Jennifer Pierce, Holistic Health Coach, JenniferPierceHealth.com*

ASK AN *expert*

Q: What are the pregnancy power foods?

A: While it's important to make sure you are eating well in general during your pregnancy (consuming adequate calories, protein, carbs, and healthy fats), there are a number of vitamins and minerals to keep in mind as well. These nutrients are not only beneficial for mom's health, but are critical for baby's growth and development for all nine months of pregnancy. Talk with your doctor about your nutrition goals regularly. Keeping a food log is a great way to stay on top of your habits and goals throughout pregnancy.

—*Stephanie L. Darby, RD LD*

TOP 10 PREGNANCY POWER NUTRIENTS[2]

NUTRIENT	BENEFIT FOR THE BABY	WHERE TO GET IT	HOW MUCH DO I NEED*
Vitamin B12	Aids in fetal brain development	All animal products, nutritional yeast	2.6 mcg/day
Vitamin D	Enhances immune function	Fish, milk, mushrooms, fortified orange juice and soy milk	15 mcg/day (600 IU)
Vitamin K	Supports bone health	Dark, leafy green vegetables	90 mcg/day
Vitamin A	Related to healthy birth weight and gestational duration	Orange and red vegetables, eggs, fish	770 mcg/day
Iodine	Aids in metabolism of proteins, carbohydrates, and fats	Iodized salt, sea products	220 mcg/day
Copper	Important for brain development and antioxidant activity	Whole grains, beans, nuts	10 mg/day
Zinc	Important for brain development	Red meat, poultry, seafood, dairy, whole grains	11 mg/day
Folate	Critical for fetal neural tube development	Dark, leafy green vegetables, legumes	400 mcg/day
Calcium	Necessary for bone growth and development	Dairy, broccoli, kale, soy foods, fortified cereals and grains	1000 mg/day
Iron	Necessary to support increased blood volume	Red meat, poultry, seafood, beans, dark, leafy greens, dried fruits, blackstrap molasses, fortified cereals and grains	27 mg/day

*Needs based on pregnant women over the age of 18.

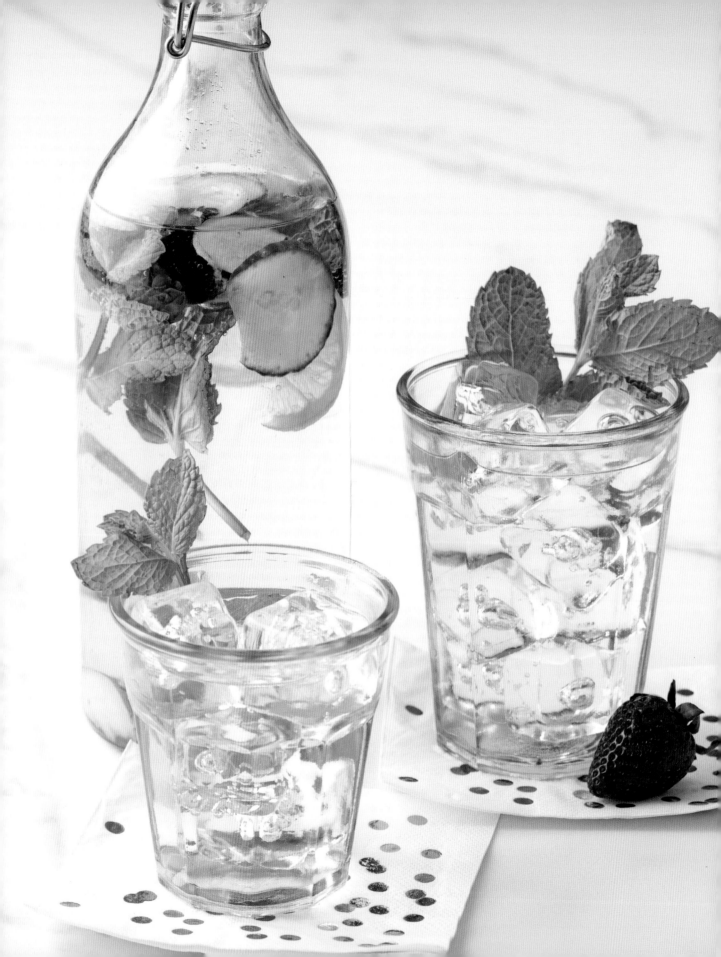

ICEBOX ELIXIR

YIELD: *About 1 quart (1 L)*

Making babies is thirsty business. It's easy to get sick of chugging down a plain clear liquid—even if it is a life-giving substance. Pregnant women are often advised to drink between 8 and 13 cups of water per day—depending on climate and body type. That's a whole lot of H_2O!

Making your daily drinking binge a little more appealing is as easy as dropping a few tasty ingredients into a pitcher. You don't even have to stir. Just pop this heavenly tincture into the refrigerator and enjoy subtly flavored water all day long.

INGREDIENTS

- 32 ounces (1 L) water
- 1 sprig fresh mint
- 2 slices ginger root, crushed
- 2 slices fresh lemon
- 2 slices cucumber, peeled

DIRECTIONS

1. Combine ingredients in a quart-sized mason jar and chill in the refrigerator for at least 30 minutes.

2. Strain and enjoy as-is or over ice.

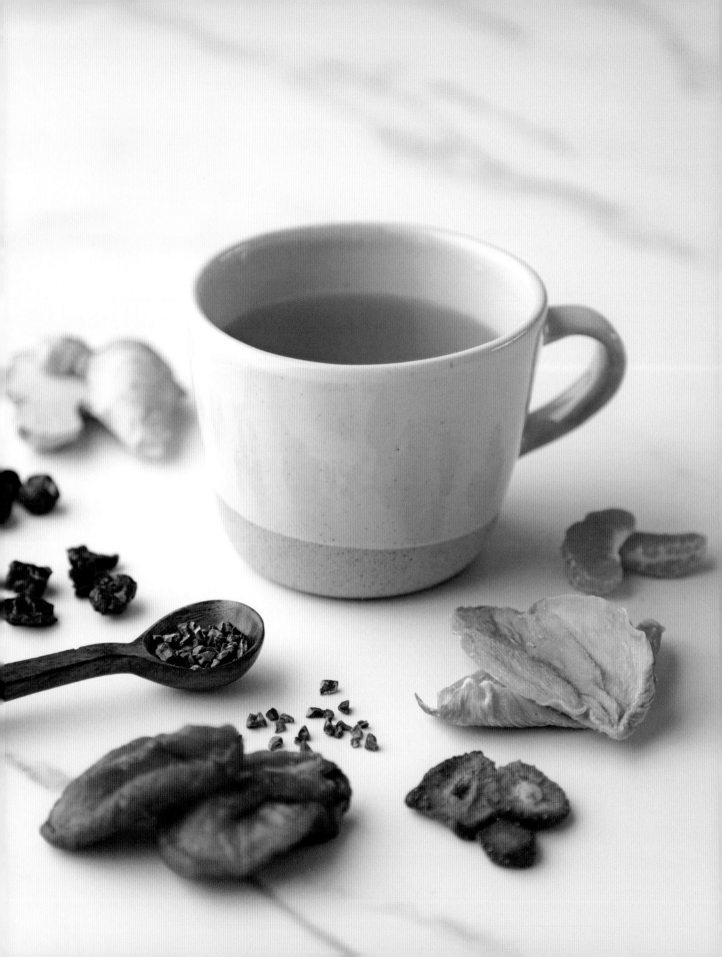

FRUIT TEAS FOR MAMA

YIELD: *About 1 cup (240 ml) each*

When my younger sister was pregnant with her first son I asked her what kind of recipes she'd want to see in a book like this. She didn't need a single moment to consider her answer. "Anything," she said, "that will make drinking all of this water a little easier!"

One easy way to mix things up is by enjoying at least one of your servings hot. Make it even better by adding some flavor. While the world of herbal tea can be tough to navigate for expecting mamas (some doctors advise against drinking *any* variety, while others permit a chosen few), fruit teas are completely safe.

They are also super easy to make and a snap to customize. Try mixing and matching flavors by substituting dried fruits, fresh citrus, fresh mint, and, of course—ginger. Add a pinch of sugar or a squirt of honey if you prefer sweet tea. You can even pour your favorite fruity brew over ice for something altogether different.

DIRECTIONS

1. Pour boiled water over ingredients and allow the tea to steep for 5 minutes. Strain solids and enjoy!

INGREDIENTS

Mango-Ginger Tea

- 1 cup (240 ml) boiled water
- 2 slices fresh ginger, crushed
- 2 tablespoons (30 ml) dried mango or apricot, diced
- 1 teaspoon (5 ml) lime juice

Cocoa-Mint Tea

- 1 cup (240 ml) boiled water
- 2 tablespoons (30 ml) fresh peppermint leaves, minced
- 1 tablespoon (15 ml) cacao nibs

Cranberry-Vanilla Tea

- 1 cup (240 ml) boiled water
- 1 tablespoon (15 ml) dried cranberries
- 2 tablespoons (30 ml) orange juice
- ¼ vanilla bean, diced

Lemon-Mint Tea

- 1 cup (240 ml) boiled water
- 2 tablespoons (30 ml) fresh peppermint leaves, minced
- 1 teaspoon (5 ml) lemon juice

Berry-Vanilla Tea

- 1 cup (240 ml) boiled water
- 1 tablespoon (15 ml) dehydrated strawberries
- 1 tablespoon (15 ml) dehydrated blueberries
- 1 teaspoon (5 ml) lemon juice
- ¼ vanilla bean, diced

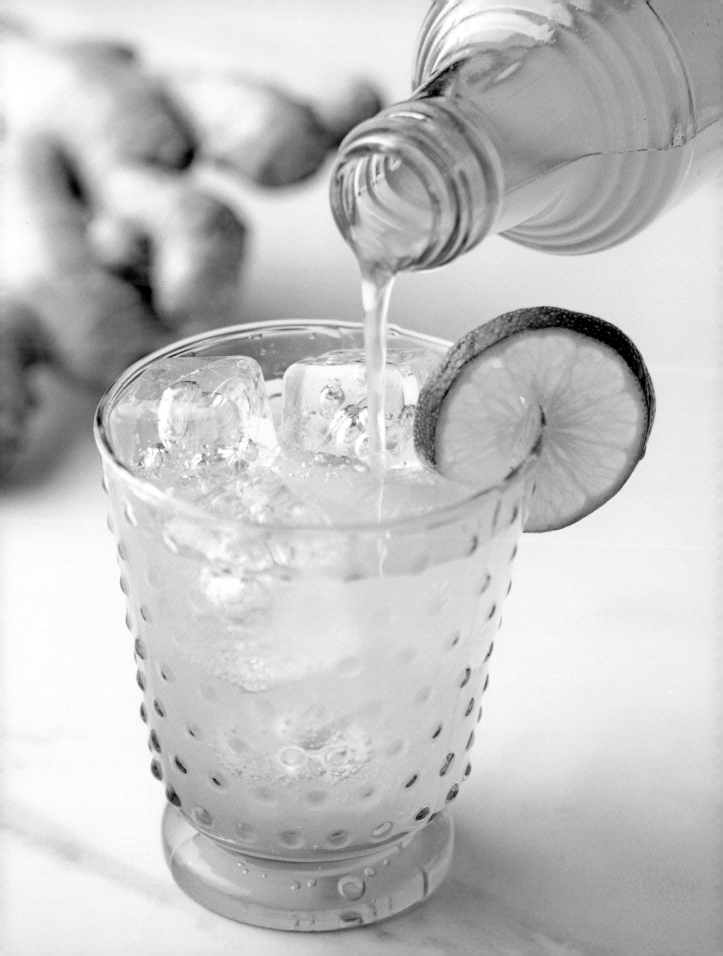

GINGER SYRUP

YIELD: *About 1 cup (240 ml)*

The term "morning sickness" ranks up there with "comfortable dress pants" in the misnomer hall of fame. They got the sickness part right, I'll give them that, but this particular malady is by no means restricted to mornings. Any mama who has felt its scourge can tell you that it's not the most pleasant part of pregnancy, but it is most certainly not confined to the beginning of the day.

Thankfully, there is a knobby little root at your grocery store that can help take the edge off your tummy troubles. Ginger has long been touted as a cure-all for weak stomachs. As someone whose father seemed to always have a can of ginger ale handy in case of a spinning roller coaster or unfortunate car trips, I can swear by its magical properties. This simple syrup makes it easy for you to add a splash (or maybe more like a swig) of ginger to any drink you like.

INGREDIENTS

- 1 cup (240 ml) turbinado (raw) sugar
- 1 cup (240 ml) water
- 2 inches of fresh ginger, peeled and grated
- 2 tablespoons (30 ml) lemon or lime juice (optional)

DIRECTIONS

1. Combine the sugar, water, and ginger in a small sauce pan. Bring the contents to a boil over high heat, then immediately reduce to a simmer.

2. Simmer for 10 minutes, until the surface of the liquid becomes thick and glossy, then remove from heat.

3. When the mixture has cooled, pour it through a fine mesh strainer. Add the lemon or lime juice if using, then mix well.

TO USE

Try adding the syrup to a pitcher of ice water, a glass of seltzer, or a cup of hot tea. You can even mix it with fruit juice to make fancy-pants mocktails or ice pops! Try starting with 1 to 3 teaspoons (5 to 15 ml) of syrup per cup (240 ml) of liquid.

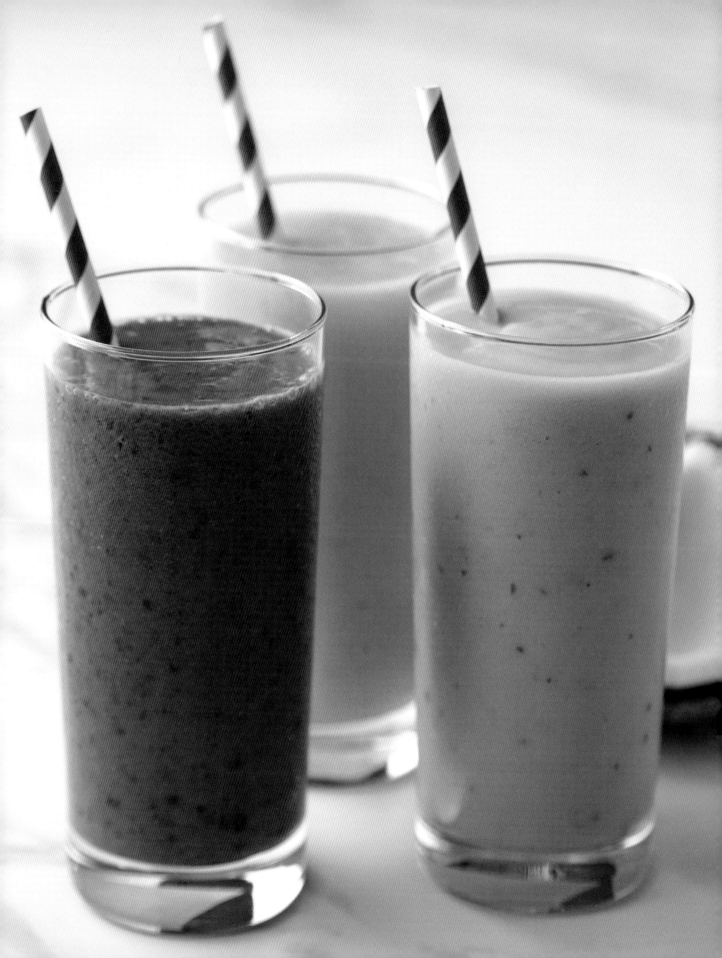

HYDRATION SMOOTHIES

YIELD: *About two 8-ounce (240 ml) servings each*

Staying hydrated can be one of the most challenging aspects of prenatal and postpartum life. It may seem like you've emptied an entire water tower all on your own by the time you reach the third trimester!

Even though they chug water all day and night, some mamas can still feel dry and experience the gut-grappling discomfort of dehydration during pregnancy and lactation. Sometimes adding a boost of nutrients (like electrolytes, antioxidants, and fatty acids) can help your body make better use of all that water. One easy (and delicious) way to do that is by making a smoothie.

Each of these recipes was created with a light, fresh flavor that isn't overly sweet or packed with sugar. You can make these smoothies your own by experimenting with different frozen fruits, flavored yogurts, or mild-tasting vegetables. You can try adding extra water, coconut water, fruit juice, or honey to adjust the texture and sweetness of the following recipes.

A little tip on smoothie-making: Always put the liquid ingredients on the bottom of the blender, followed by the soft, and then the frozen ingredients. This helps everything blend as smoothly as possible.

INGREDIENTS

Berry-Watermelon Smoothie

- ½ cup (120 ml) coconut water
- 2 cups (480 ml) frozen berries
- 1 cup (240 ml) fresh seedless watermelon, diced
- ½ cup (120 ml) plain or vanilla-flavored yogurt

Cucumber-Avocado Smoothie

- ¾ cup (180 ml) coconut water
- 1 tablespoon (15 ml) lime juice
- ½ cup (120 ml) ripe avocado
- 1 cup (240 ml) cucumber, peeled and diced
- 1 cup (240 ml) frozen pineapple

Mango-Ginger Smoothie

- ½ cup (120 ml) coconut water
- 1 cup (240 ml) frozen mango
- ½ banana, sliced
- ½ cup (120 ml) yellow bell pepper, diced
- ½ teaspoon (2.5 ml) fresh ginger, peeled and grated

DIRECTIONS

1. Place any liquid ingredients into the bottom of the blender first, followed by the fresh ingredients. Place the frozen ingredients into the blender last.

2. Secure the top of the blender, then blend at a slow speed for 30 seconds. Increase to a high speed and blend for 2 more minutes.

3. If the smoothie ends up being too thick or chunky to blend easily, try adding 1 or 2 tablespoons of water or coconut water, then blending again.

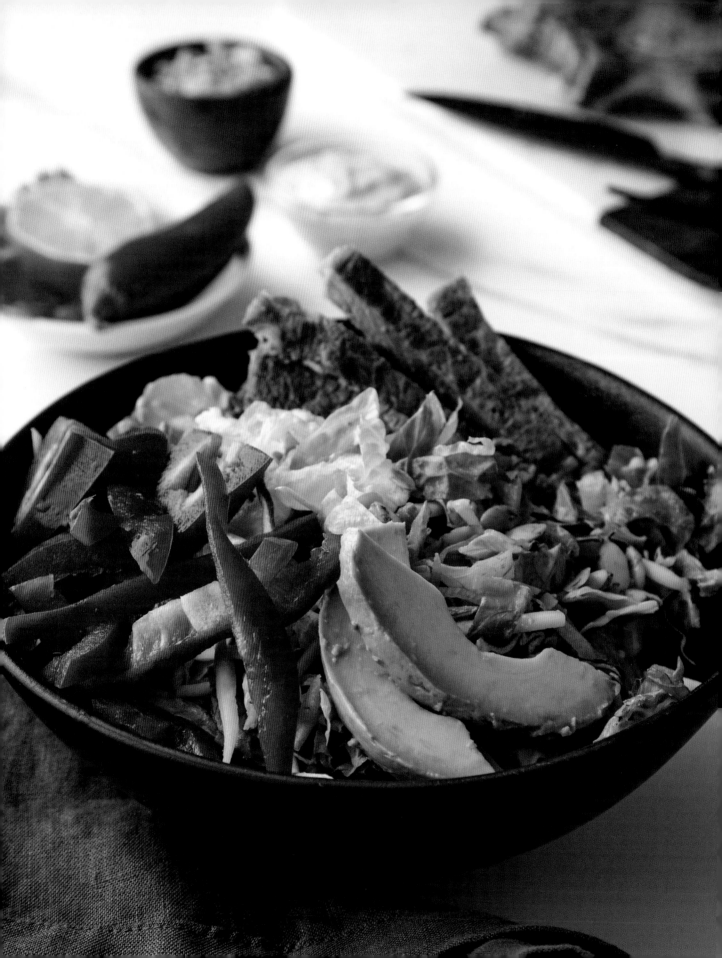

IRON WOMAN CHOPPED SALAD

YIELD: *2½ cups (600 ml) (1 serving)*

One of the best things you can do for your body while it is growing another human being is keep it well fed. Baby will be working hard to absorb as many vitamins and nutrients as possible during his or her forty-week stay and it can sometimes be challenging to keep up with your body's demand for essential vitamins and minerals.

Hearty salads like this one can make getting the nutrition you need a downright pleasurable experience. Loaded with dark, leafy greens, fresh peppers and carrots, and crunchy pumpkin seeds, this is a satisfying way to load up on goodies like iron, vitamin C, and folate.

Chopping the greens into small bites makes them less chewy and easier to enjoy—even if you aren't particularly fond of kale. (The kale and cabbage can also be swapped out for more tender greens such as baby spinach or arugula, if that's more to your liking.) I've included two dressings for this salad. The first one is rich, creamy, and just a little spicy. The second is a simple balsamic vinaigrette. Switching up the dressing is a great way to keep this recipe interesting enough to enjoy over and over. You can also substitute your own favorite dressing for yet another option.

Try topping this salad with grilled chicken, steak, tofu, or a fried egg to add protein and make it even more filling.

INGREDIENTS

- ½ cup (120 ml) kale, stems and spines removed, shredded
- ½ cup (120 ml) romaine lettuce, shredded
- ½ cup (120 ml) cabbage, shredded
- ¼ cup (60 ml) carrots, shredded
- ¼ cup (60 ml) red bell pepper, diced
- ¼ cup (60 ml) raw or toasted pumpkin seeds
- ¼ cup (60 ml) avocado, diced (about ½ avocado)
- 2 tablespoons (30 ml) salad dressing (see recipes on page 78)

DIRECTIONS

1. Rub the shredded kale between your palms to give it a quick massage. This will make the kale more tender and easier to chew.

2. Combine the kale with the lettuce, cabbage, carrots, and bell pepper in a bowl and toss to combine.

3. Top with seeds, avocado, and salad dressing.

INGREDIENTS

- » ¼ cup (60 ml) mayonnaise or plain Greek yogurt
- » ¼ cup (60 ml) chopped cilantro
- » ¼ cup (60 ml) avocado (about ½ avocado)
- » 1 tablespoon jalapeno, minced (optional)
- » 2 tablespoons (30 ml) lime juice (1 to 2 limes)
- » 2 tablespoons (30 ml) virgin olive oil
- » ¼ teaspoon (1.25 ml) salt
- » ⅛ teaspoon (0.75 ml) black pepper

Creamy Cilantro Lime Dressing

YIELD: *About ½ cup (120 ml)*

DIRECTIONS

1. Combine all ingredients in a blender or food processor and puree until smooth.
2. If needed, add water, 1 teaspoon at a time, to yield a smooth texture.
3. Refrigerate for up to 10 days.

INGREDIENTS

- » 1 teaspoon (5 ml) Dijon mustard
- » 1 teaspoon (5 ml) ketchup
- » 1 teaspoon (5 ml) honey
- » ¼ cup (60 ml) balsamic vinegar
- » ½ cup (120 ml) virgin olive oil
- » ¼ teaspoon (1.25 ml) salt
- » ⅛ teaspoon (0.75 ml) black pepper

Balsamic Vinaigrette Dressing

YIELD: *About ¾ cup (180 ml)*

DIRECTIONS

1. Whisk together the mustard, ketchup, honey, and vinegar in a small bowl until well blended.
2. While whisking continuously, drizzle the olive oil into the bowl in a slow, steady stream.
3. Add salt and pepper, then whisk again.
4. Refrigerate for up to 1 month.

HEAT & EAT RICE BOWLS

YIELD: *About 1¾ cups (415 ml) (1 serving)*

Did I mention that staying well fed was a really great thing to do for your body, both during pregnancy and the postpartum period? Well, it is. That's no surprise really, but neither is the fact that keeping up with a healthy diet can be really challenging. Juggling family responsibilities, work commitments, ever-changing finances, and fatigue from growing and then living with a new baby can leave very little time to cook. Heck, it can leave very little time to eat!

Preparing foods you can heat and toss over healthy grains is an excellent strategy. By cooking your main ingredients ahead of time, you'll be able to throw together quick meals that will nourish your body without requiring a whole lot of time or attention. I suggest picking one of each of the main ingredient categories below to prepare once a week.

Stock your fridge with several ready-to-eat flavor boosters and a variety of sauces and seasonings so that you can add some variety to your week of meals. Try a different combination of grains, protein, and vegetables the next week and you'll have a whole new menu to explore!

For more ideas and complete recipes on how to prepare the suggestions below, visit https://tinyurl.com/RiceBowlsEBook and download your own free copy of my companion e-cookbook, *Mary Makes Good: Heat & Eat Rice Bowls.*

MAIN INGREDIENTS

See directions at left and make-ahead instructions on pages 81 and 82

Flavor Boosters

- Avocado
- Diced or shredded cheese
- Hummus
- Seaweed or furikake seasoning
- Raw or toasted sesame or pumpkin seeds

Sauces & Seasonings

- Sour cream or Greek yogurt
- Sriracha sauce
- Japanese mayo
- Soy sauce, tamari, or liquid aminos
- Lime or lemon juice
- Olive, flax seed, avocado, or coconut oil

DIRECTIONS

1. Ahead of time, prepare one food from each of the following categories as indicated: cooked grain (page 81), protein (page 81), and green and red/orange vegetables (page 82).

2. Warm ½ cup grain, ¼ cup protein, and ½ cup each green and red/orange veggies according to preference; place in bowl.

3. Top with 1 to 2 tablespoons flavor boosters and 1 to 3 teaspoons sauces or seasonings to taste (shown at above).

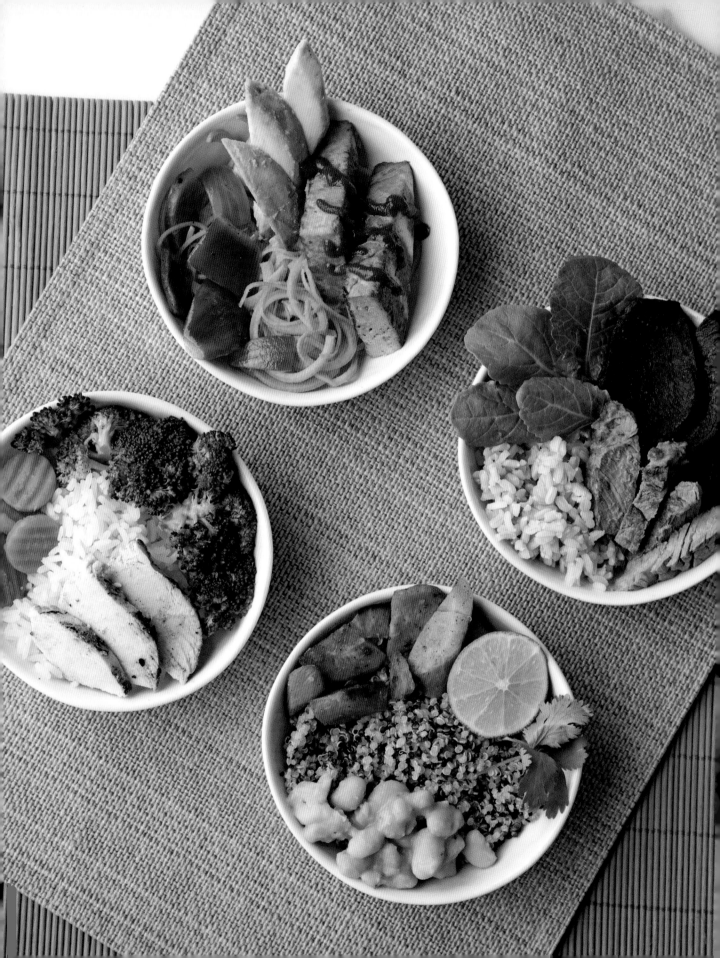

HEAT & EAT RICE BOWLS *(continued)*

Cooking Methods for Grains (Pick One)

Brown rice
Combine 1 cup rice with 1½ cups water and ¼ teaspoon salt in saucepan. Bring to boil. Reduce to simmer and cover. Cook on low heat for 20 minutes. Turn off heat and let rice sit, covered, for 10–20 minutes. (10 minutes = al dente; 20 minutes = tender)

Basmati rice
Soak 1 cup rice in cold water for 30 minutes. Drain rice and rinse twice, or until the water runs clear. Combine rice with 1¾ cup cold water and ¼ teaspoon salt in a saucepan. Bring water to boil, reduce to simmer, cover, and cook on low for 20 minutes. Turn off heat and let rice sit, covered, for 5 minutes.

Wild rice
Rinse ½ cup wild rice with cold water. Combine rice with 2 cups cold water or broth and ¼ teaspoon salt in saucepan. Bring to boil, then reduce to simmer, cover, and cook on low heat until tender (45–60 minutes).

Quinoa
Rinse 1 cup quinoa with cold water. Combine quinoa with 2 cups cold water and ¼ teaspoon salt in a saucepan. Bring water to boil, reduce to simmer, cover, and cook on low for 15–20 minutes. (15 minutes = firm; 20 minutes = soft)

Cauliflower rice
Shred raw florets with grater or food processor. Heat large skillet with 1 tablespoon cooking oil. Saute for 5 minutes or until tender.

Cooking Methods for Proteins (Pick One)

Chickpeas
Canned: Rinse and heat.
Dried: Soak and boil according to package directions.

Beans
Canned: Rinse and heat.
Dried: Soak and boil according to package directions.

Lentils
Prepare according to package directions.

Tofu
Marinate 24 hours, then fry in cast iron pan until edges are crisp.

Eggs
Fry, scramble, or hard boil.

Beef
Roast, grill, saute, or braise to an internal temperature of 145°F (63°C).

Pork
Roast, grill, saute, or braise to an internal temperature of 145°F (63°C).

Chicken
Roast, grill, saute, poach, or braise to an internal temperature of 165°F (74°C).

Fish
Roast, grill, saute, or braise to an internal temperature of 145°F (63°C).

HEAT & EAT RICE BOWLS *(continued)*

PREP FOR GREEN VEGGIES (PICK ONE)

VEGGIES	RAW	ROASTED WITH SPLASH OF OIL AT 400°F (204°C)	STEAMED
Kale	Shredded	15–20 minutes	4–5 minutes
Baby spinach	Whole		1–2 minutes
Broccoli	Shredded	15–20 minutes	4–5 minutes
Arugula	Whole		1–2 minutes
Green beans	Diced		4–5 minutes
Brussel sprouts	Shredded	35–45 minutes	6–8 minutes
Green peas			10–15 minutes if raw / 4–5 minutes if frozen

PREP FOR RED/ORANGE VEGGIES (PICK ONE)

VEGGIES	RAW	ROASTED WITH SPLASH OF OIL AT 400°F (204°C)	STEAMED
Sweet potato		Diced, 40–50 minutes	Diced, 15–20 minutes
Carrot	Shredded or spiralized	20 minutes	7–10 minutes
Butternut squash		Diced, 30 minutes	Diced, 10–15 minutes
Beets	Shredded or spiralized	Diced, 35–40 minutes	Diced, 10–20 minutes

MAMA BARS: THE ULTIMATE POSTPARTUM COOKIE

YIELD: *About 24 bars*

As a cornerstone of any well-rounded postpartum diet, the all-mighty postpartum cookie provides nutritional support to mamas during baby's first few months and beyond. Birthing and raising a baby is exhausting business. Though often called lactation cookies, these hearty little treats can provide quick, enjoyable sustenance to both nursing and bottle-feeding mamas.

This cookie starts off with a classic sugar, flour, and butter base, with a dose of iron-rich molasses. Whole oats, flax seeds, hemp hearts, brewer's yeast, and almond flour give the cookies a rich array of protein and nutrients. Dark chocolate chips are added for sheer pleasure. If you prefer, try swapping out the chocolate for raisins or another type of dried fruit.

I jokingly forbade my husband to eat these because he was neither lactating nor postpartum, but these cookies do make an awesome snack for anyone helping to care for baby during those early months (or years). Be sure to make and freeze extra so there will be plenty for Daddy, Grandma, Auntie, and anyone else who is down there in the trenches with you.

I opted to make these into bars instead of traditional drop cookies, seeing as they were exceptionally thick and hearty. Plus, to me, a bar feels a little less like a dessert and a little more like a power food—which these certainly qualify for. If you don't have a 4-quart (10 x 15-inch) baking dish handy, or if you just prefer a more classic cookie shape, simply drop the dough in 2-tablespoon dollops onto a baking sheet lined with parchment paper to form drop cookies.

INGREDIENTS

- 2 tablespoons (30 ml) ground flax seed
- ¼ cup (60 ml) water
- 1 cup (240 ml) unsalted butter, softened
- 1 cup (240 ml) sugar
- ⅓ cup (80 ml) light brown sugar
- 2 eggs
- ⅓ cup (80 ml) blackstrap molasses
- 1 teaspoon (5 ml) vanilla extract
- 2¼ cups (540 ml) whole wheat flour or gluten-free flour (recipe page 30)
- ¼ cup (60 ml) almond flour/meal
- ¼ cup (60 ml) hemp hearts, hulled
- ¼ cup (60 ml) brewer's yeast
- 1 teaspoon (5 ml) salt
- 1 teaspoon (5 ml) baking soda
- 1 teaspoon (5 ml) cinnamon
- 2 cups (480 ml) old-fashioned oats
- 1 cup (240 ml) dark chocolate chips or chopped dried fruit

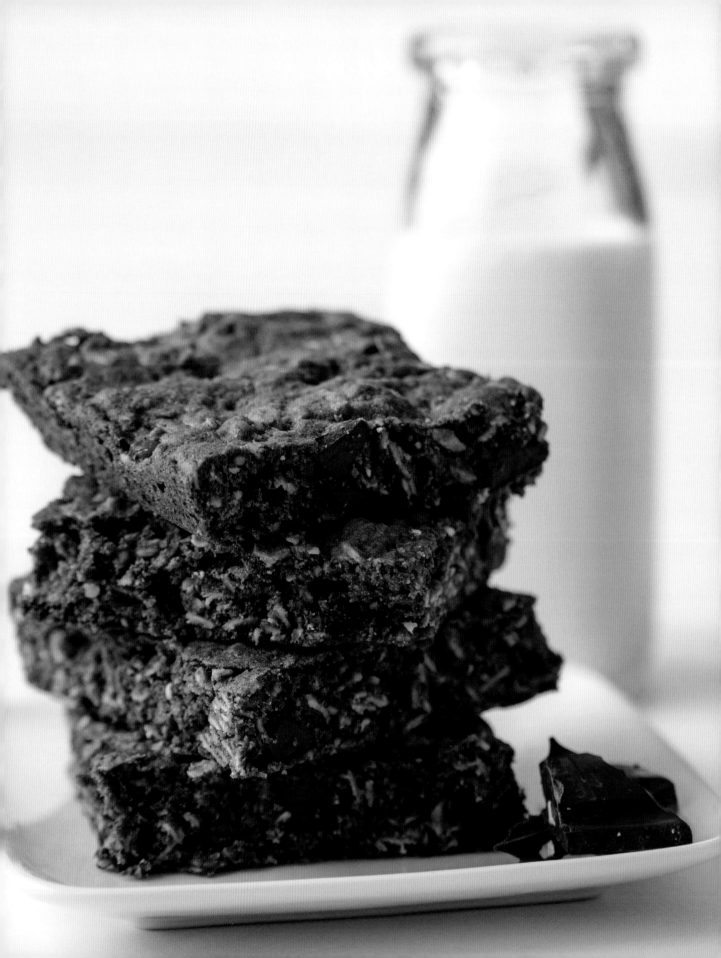

MAMA BARS *(continued)*

DIRECTIONS

1. Preheat the oven to 350°F (177°C).

2. Combine the flax seeds and water in a small bowl and set aside.

3. Cream the butter and sugars together in the bowl of an electric stand mixer fitted with the paddle attachment. Beat for 10 minutes or until fluffy.

4. Add the soaked flax seeds with water, eggs, molasses, and vanilla and mix until well blended. (Scrape the sides down before blending to make sure everything mixes evenly.)

5. In a separate bowl, whisk together the whole wheat or gluten-free flour, almond flour/meal, hemp hearts, brewer's yeast, salt, baking soda, and cinnamon.

6. Add the dry ingredients to the wet in two parts. Mix until just combined.

7. Add the oats and chocolate chips or dried fruit with the mixer on a slow speed. Mix until just combined.

8. Line a 10 x 15-inch (4 quart) baking dish with parchment paper. Drop the dough into the dish and do your best to spread it evenly across the dish so that it is touching each side and corner. It's okay if it's a bit lumpy or uneven.

9. Bake the bars for about 30 minutes or until the edges of the dough become deep golden brown and the dough in the middle of the pan appears to be thoroughly baked. Rotate the pan about halfway through cooking. If using gluten-free flour, bake for an additional 10 to 15 minutes.

10. Remove the dish from the oven and allow to cool for 1 hour before slicing into bars. Fully cooled bars can be frozen for up to 3 months in airtight packaging.

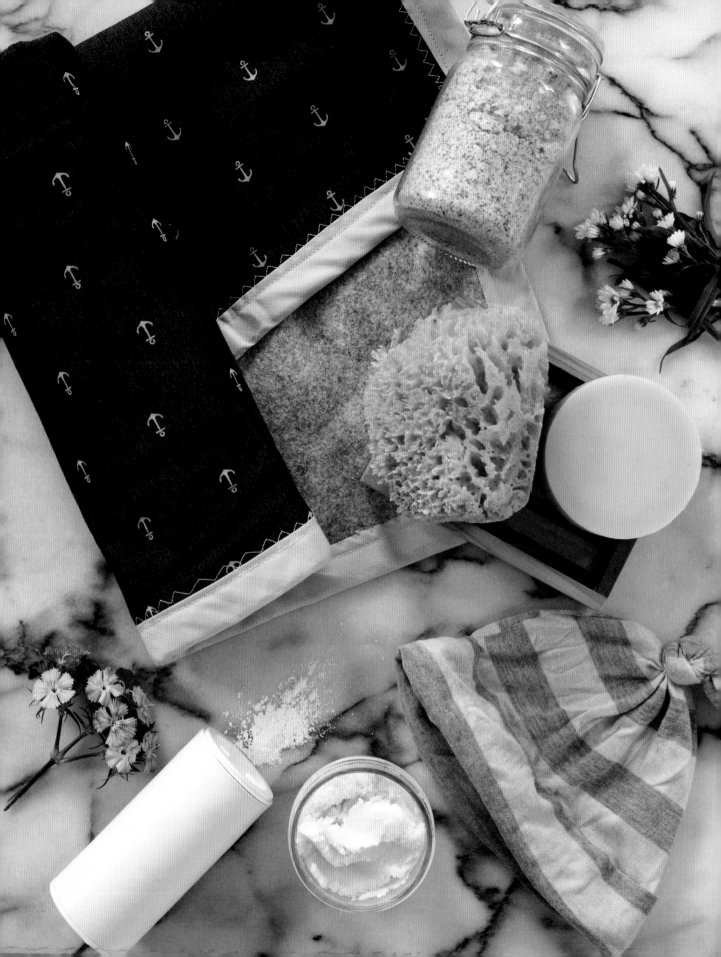

chapter 3

BABY BATH & BODY

That new baby smell—it's pretty intoxicating, right? You nuzzle your face into the soft, fuzzy down on top of a baby's head, and *pow,* your heart is fluttering like a hummingbird on a honeysuckle. My son's head smelled like warm sugar cookies—a combination of sweet milk, baby sweat, and something mysteriously toasty that I will probably never identify (but hopefully never forget). I don't know if this is true for all mothers, but I feel like I could have picked that smell out blindfolded with no problem at all. Even now, as he grows from a toddler into a little kid, I can still detect an undertone of his newborn scent beneath his curls.

I can't imagine why anyone would feel the need to cover the magical aroma of a brand-new baby with perfumes and synthetic fragrances. It's just unnecessary. Babies look and smell just fine as they are and require very little in the way of "beauty" products. As long as you have something simple to wash them with (plain water works surprisingly well, actually) and something to soothe their skin when it is dry or irritated, you are good to go! →

allergies, sensitivities, and baby care

If your child is suffering from persistent rashes or irritation, you may be observing a sensitivity to an ingredient in baby's skin care products. Even natural ingredients can sometimes disagree with our skin—especially when that skin is brand new and ultra sensitive! Performing a patch test is an easy way to determine whether your child is sensitive to a particular ingredient or skin care product.

Please note that patch tests should never be used to diagnose dangerous allergies. If your family has a history of allergic reactions or you suspect your child might have an allergy (as opposed to a sensitivity, which is mild in comparison) consult your doctor before trying any ingredient that is related to that allergen.

Some examples of skin care ingredients that relate to potentially dangerous allergens and *should not* be patch tested*:

⇒ Soybean oil (soy)
⇒ Peanut oil (peanuts)
⇒ Almond oil (tree nuts)
⇒ Shea butter (latex)
⇒ Whole oats (gluten)

*Do not perform patch tests with these ingredients. Talk to your doctor about how to safely diagnose allergies.

HOW TO PERFORM A PATCH TEST

1. Start by cleaning baby's skin with warm water.

2. Pick an inconspicuous spot on baby, such as the lower leg or upper arm, and apply a dab of the ingredient. (Please note that undiluted essential oils should never be applied directly to the skin.)

3. Watch the spot where the ingredient was applied for twenty four to forty eight hours to see if any rash or redness develops.

4. If signs of sensitivity occur, consult your pediatrician to see if further allergy testing is needed.

a newborn's perfectly imperfect skin

"They are so perfect!" You'll find yourself and others making similar exclamations upon examining tiny fingers, miniature toes, and the impossibly soft skin of your newborn baby. While your baby is surely just as he should be, the description of "perfect" might be slightly misleading. For example, it is *perfectly* normal for newborns to experience acne, rashes, cradle cap, peeling skin, and milia. Your baby may even develop little white spots or big red blotches.

This can be pretty alarming, but fear not! Your perfect baby is just getting comfortable in his or her own skin. That's not always a pretty process. Most babies grow out of these mild skin conditions within the first few months with little to no intervention. As always, if something really has you worried, looks infected, or has lasted longer than a week, don't hesitate to consult your doctor. There may be something you can do to make your little one more comfortable, or at least ease your own worries.

CRADLE CAP

Cradle cap is similar in look and nature to dandruff, showing up as a hard, scaly, crustlike coating on baby's head. While cradle cap can be unsightly and a pain to deal with, it is incredibly common and usually resolves itself as baby grows older. You can help it along with the Oatmeal Scrub on page 102, or ask your pediatrician and mama friends for tips on how they tackled it with their own kids.

ECZEMA

This is one of those words that gets applied to a range of mild to moderate skin conditions. It is usually used to name patches of very dry, itchy, or red skin. Often, a petroleum-based ointment is advised, and in some cases, it's the only thing that does the trick. If you'd like to try a more natural alternative first, reach for the Herbal Body Oil on page 26, or try a whole ingredient like cocoa butter, castor oil, or apricot kernel oil.

RINGWORM

This one sounds pretty awful, but really, it's just a common fungal infection with no worms involved at all. The rash gets its name from its appearance. It often shows up as a bright red circle—but not always. Ringworm can also just appear as a really nasty diaper rash. You might need your doctor's help to pinpoint what kind of fungus you are dealing with and how best to treat it. A prescription or over-the-counter medication is likely to be necessary to clear up a case of ringworm, but in some cases, antifungal oils like neem oil or karanja can help too.

mama mana: the magical and mysterious power of breastmilk

Baby has acne? Apply a little breast milk. Is your little one's skin looking dry, red, or itchy? Mommy milk to the rescue. Did baby try to scratch up his or her gorgeous face? You guessed it. Breast milk can help! Mamas have been taking advantage of the amazing restorative powers of breast milk ever since mamas and babies

---

Additive Alert

SODIUM LAURYL SULFATE

SLS (sodium lauryl sulfate) is a detergent commonly added to liquid soaps, bubble bath, and shampoo. This ingredient helps create the big fluffy suds and bubbles that people love in commercial products. Unfortunately, it can also be seriously irritating to sensitive skin. Babies may have a hard time dealing with the presence of SLS or other sulfate-based detergents in their skin care products.

existed—which is the entire history of mankind. You can use it to soothe baby's skin and to heal your own chapped skin. It can even be used as an ingredient in skin care recipes like lotions, creams, and cold-process soaps!

adding essential oils

Essential oils are extremely potent plant extracts that can be used in the practice of aromatherapy and holistic and herbal medicine. They are so potent that they can be used just like medicine. And like medicines, they need to be used with extreme caution when it comes to babies and kids.

While there are essential oils that can be used with babies and young children at a low dilution (usually around 0.1 to 0.5% of a total product), there are others that can cause toxicity, seizures, and other very serious injuries. Peppermint, for example, should never be used with a child under the age of two.

The following chart includes four essential oils that are commonly used on babies and toddlers over six months of age without incident. However, it's important to remember that these are highly potent substances with powerful properties and the results of using them isn't always predictable. To learn more about essential oil safety, visit The National Association for Holistic Aromatherapy's Web site at naha.org.

If you or your child have any health conditions, or if your child is under six

ASK AN *expert*

Q: How often should I bathe my baby?

A: According to the American Academy of Pediatrics, it is perfectly appropriate to bathe your baby no more than two to three times a week, and focus on daily cleansing of dirty areas (hands, knees, feet, diaper area, face), rather than a daily immersion bath, as your baby becomes more mobile and starts to eat solids. Skin folds should be frequently monitored for redness or irritation and spot-cleaned as necessary.

—*Dr. Suzanne Van Benthuysen, MD, FAAP, IBCLC, beewellaustin.com*

months old, I urge you to consult your pediatrician before using any essential oils, even those listed here. If you do decide to add essential oils to the skin or hair care recipes in this chapter, be sure to follow the usage rates indicated here. Keep in mind that an overdose of essential oil has the potential to seriously harm your child.

sun block

For babies under six months old, the best protection from sun damage is simply limiting exposure to direct sunlight. After baby reaches six months, you can begin applying sunscreen to help keep skin safe. When it comes to protecting baby's skin from sun damage, it's best to stick to professionally manufactured products. While there are many natural ingredients that contain elements that can help stop sun damage, it's impossible to know exactly how much sun protection a homemade recipe will offer. Sun Protection Factor (SPF) values are determined using sophisticated lab testing. In fact, it's against FDA regulations to market a product as containing SPF value without those tests having been run.

That being said, not all sun care products are created equal. For the healthiest choice possible, make a habit of reading the back of the bottle and scrutinizing ingredients. For starters, seek out natural products that don't contain paraben preservatives, synthetic dyes, and artificial fragrances. Opt for a high SPF value (50 or higher) and look for sunscreens that have been formulated specifically for infants and children. Whatever brand you choose, be sure to apply sunscreen often. Unprotected exposure can lead to premature aging, skin damage, and even cancer.

The Environmental Working Group offers an annual guide to shopping for the safest and most effective brands of sunscreen. Find their latest recommendations at ewg.org.

insect repellent

Choosing the right insect repellent for babies and small children can be a tricky decision for any parent—especially for parents who are concerned about exposure to synthetic chemicals. For the first six months of baby's life, the best protection is limiting a child's exposure to biting insects. Mosquito netting can be used to shield strollers and cribs, and dressing babies in long sleeves and pants can help too. When children reach around six months of age, most pediatricians will recommend starting the use of insect repellent.

ESSENTIAL OILS COMMONLY USED IN BABY AND CHILD CARE

ESSENTIAL OIL	SCIENTIFIC NAME	PROPERTIES
Roman Chamomile	*Anthemis nobilis*	Anti-inflammatory, calming, soothing
Lavender	*Lavandula angustifolia*	Anti-bacterial, balancing
Sandalwood	*Santalum spicatum*	Balancing, calming, soothing
Sweet Orange	*Citrus sinensis*	Anti-bacterial, uplifting

The following have these usage rates for babies six months and older:
General usage rate of 0.25–0.5% / 3–5 drops of essential oil per ounce of carrier oil
Diapering Ointments: Up to 30 drops
Herbal Body Oil: Up to 40 drops
All-Over Baby Wash: Up to 16 drops
Oatmeal Scrub: Not recommended

Synthetic repellents that include ingredients like DEET or Picaridin are proven to be highly effective, but not everyone is comfortable with using them on small kids. Natural alternatives that use essential oils and plant extracts are sometimes less effective, but have the appeal of being plant based.

Speak to your pediatrician about making the right choice for your family. Your risk of insect-born illness may vary depending on your location and lifestyle. If you do choose a natural repellent, make sure that any essential oils used are safe for your child's age group. You can learn more about essential oil safety for babies and kids on The National Association for Holistic Aromatherapy's Web site (naha.org).

soft & simple baby massage

Mama's touch can be a powerful thing. The gentle pressure and skin-to-skin contact provided by the simple practice of baby massage can help to soothe babies, provide valuable sensory input, and even assist digestion. My favorite oil for baby massage is apricot kernel oil. This everyday nourishing oil is even better when infused with helpful herbs. Look for the Herbal Body Oil on page 26 for the ultimate baby massage oil.

A soft and gentle touch is all that's needed when massaging a baby.

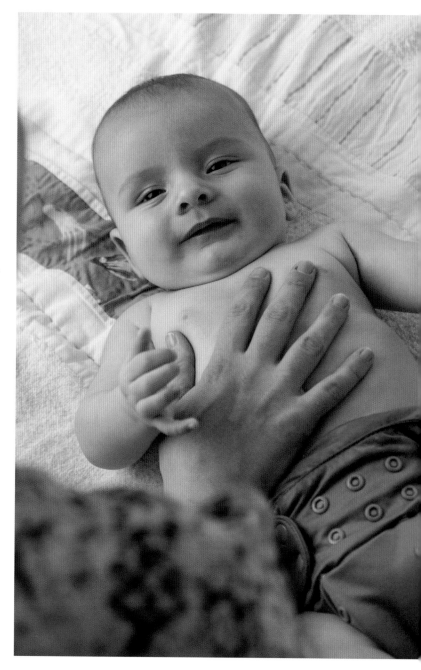

The younger an infant is, the lighter the pressure that is appropriate. To get started, place baby on a safe, comfortable surface, like a crib or changing table. Drizzle a few drops of massage oil into the palm of your hand and rub your hands together to warm the oil.

Gently open baby's palms and rub them with your thumbs, then glide your hands down baby's arms. Repeat this motion a few times before moving on to the feet and legs, which you will massage in a similar fashion.

Use a light touch to stroke baby's back and belly, allowing the weight of your hands to apply all the pressure needed. Baby massage is much more about touch than it is about pressure. When you are finished with the massage, pick baby up and have a nice snuggle. You should both feel pretty cozy by then.

cloth diapering 101

Babies can go through a whole lot of diapers during their infant years. Cloth diapers provide an environmentally friendly alternative to disposable diapers and they can also save moms and dads a small fortune in the long run.

If that's not a good enough incentive for you, think about what disposable diapers are made of. These little bundles of plastic are laden with synthetic chemicals—some with pretty dicey reputations. Dioxin and TBT (tributyltin) are two particularly nasty chemicals with possible links to serious health problems like hormone disruption and cancer.

Using cloth diapers does require a little extra work and know-how, but once you get into the habit, cloth diapering really is no big deal. Cloth diapers usually involve two parts: an insert to catch the goods and a cover to keep them contained. Though the premise is simple, in practice the variety of cloth diapers are surprisingly different. Little things, like snaps versus hook-and-loop tape, or PUL fabric versus wool, leave a lot of room for personal preference. I recommend checking out a few different kinds in person before investing in a set of diapers.

TYPES OF CLOTH DIAPERS

» **Prefold.** These are the classic rectangular diapers many of us used as babies before disposable diapers were an everyday thing. They are very absorbent, but not waterproof, so are typically used with a diaper cover.

» **Contour.** These are similar to prefold diapers, but cleverly curved to make folding easier. These are also typically used with diaper covers.

» **Fitted, Pocket, and All-in-One.** There are several brands available that make readymade systems of cloth diaper covers and matching inserts. These vary in style, materials, choice of fastener, and in how the insert is situated within the diaper.

⇒ **Diaper Covers.** These must be used along with an insert such as a prefold or a contour diaper. Covers are made from waterproof or water-resistant material, such as PUL, wool, or fleece.

TIPS FOR USING CLOTH DIAPERS

⇒ **Invest in a wet bag.** A wet bag is a reusable waterproof bag to hold soiled diapers. It's good to have two large ones for the nursery and two or three small ones for the diaper bag.

⇒ **Change baby often.** Cloth diapers don't wick moisture away as effectively as disposable diapers, so babies will need to be changed a little more often—ideally as soon as diapers have been soiled.

⇒ **Don't wash the doody.** Always remove solid waste from the diaper and flush it down the toilet before washing. Getting a diaper sprayer attachment on your toilet can be a big help.

ASK AN *expert*

Q: When will my baby sleep through the night?

A: Sleep deprivation is one of the most challenging aspects of new parenthood, but frequent nighttime waking keeps newborns safe and well fed. Most babies do not begin sleeping through the night without waking until about three months of age, or at twelve to thirteen pounds. Sleep issues should be addressed individually with your child's care provider or with an infant sleep specialist, especially if your baby is not gaining weight or feeding adequately, or if sleep deprivation is impairing your ability to safely care for yourself or your child.

—*Dr. Suzanne Van Benthuysen, MD, FAAP, IBCLC, beewellaustin.com*

⇒ **Don't use fabric softeners or dryer sheets.** These products can reduce absorbency and make diapers less effective.

⇒ **Invest in a diaper-safe laundry detergent.** Not all laundry detergents can clean cloth diapers effectively. Some types can even leave residue that makes them less absorbent or more prone to lingering odors. For a list of recommended detergents, check out fluffloveuniversity.com.

sweet & cuddly co-bathing

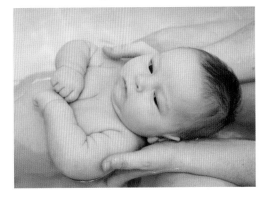

I was a little nervous about the whole thing. What if I dropped him? What if I slipped? What if my nudity somehow traumatized him? These were my thoughts as I filled up the tub, but as soon as Charlie's little feet touched the water, my fears were erased. His face broke into a huge smile—a look of utter joy. As I eased him into the bath, he squealed and squawked in delight. Once his body was submerged he began to float, then to wriggle—as if he wanted to just swim away.

I gave him as much freedom as I could while keeping a firm grip and his head above water. He kicked and splashed—totally at home in this little wet world. When we were done, we dried off, dressed, and nursed. I held him in my arms and realized that having him was the best choice I ever made.

I wanted a baby for so long, and often when we want things so intensely, we are let down when we finally get them—the reality never quite living up to the dream. It's not like that with him. Not at all. When it comes to being a mother, the reality left my dream in the dust. I hope I never forget the way he smiled that night, or the way his little face reassured me. It was like he was saying "It's okay, Mama. I know how to do this."

When I stop and think about it, I guess he's been telling me that all along.

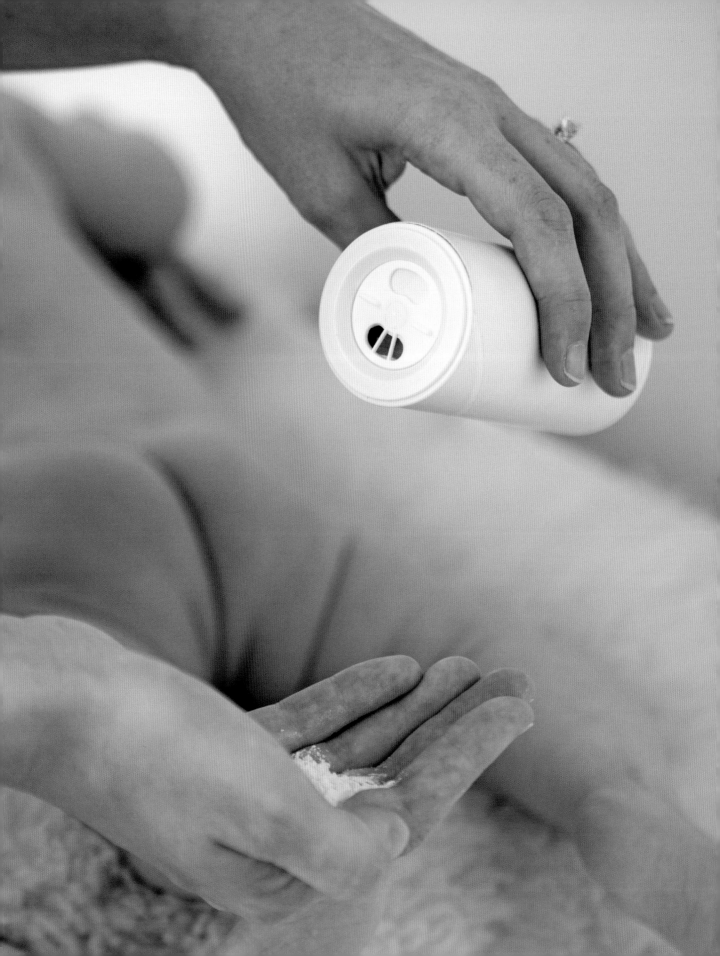

BABY POWDER

Yield: 1 cup (240 ml)

've always been a big fan of chubby babies, the pudgier the better! But all that darling chub comes with a price—things can get awfully funky between those rolls. Keeping baby's skin clean and dry can be an ongoing battle, and a good baby powder can help make the task a whole lot easier.

Commercial baby powder is often made of talc, a surprisingly nasty ingredient linked to all kinds of horrible health issues—even cancer! You can find talc-free powders from fancy-pants baby brands, but making your own is relatively cheap and easy using just a few simple ingredients.

INGREDIENTS

- ½ cup (120 ml) white kaolin clay
- ¼ cup (60 ml) oat starch
- ¼ cup (60 ml) arrowroot powder

DIRECTIONS

1. Whisk ingredients together, then pour them carefully into a jar or powder sifter.

2. Store in a dry place at room temperature for up to 1 year.

TO USE

Tap a small amount into the palm of your hand, then carefully rub it onto baby's skin. Avoid baby's eyes, nose, and mouth.

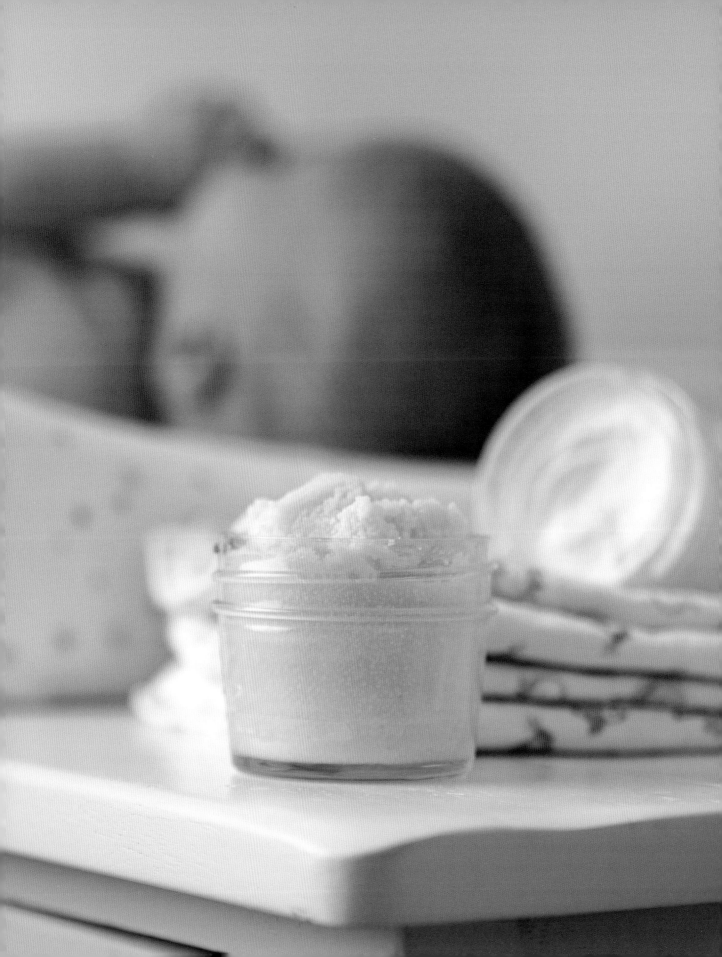

DIAPERING OINTMENTS

Yield: About 12 ounces (360 ml)

Whether you choose cloth or disposable diapers, your little one's tushy is bound to suffer the occasional rash or irritation. Exposure to constant moisture would leave anyone's skin feeling crabby, but when the party really gets started down below, the combination of substances in baby's diaper can actually create an acidic environment that can burn baby's skin!

I've seen some gnarly diaper rashes over the years, and one thing that can help both prevent and soothe such rashes is a good diapering ointment. Unlike regular balms and moisturizers that are formulated to sink into the skin quickly, diapering ointment is designed to sit on top of baby's skin, creating a barrier between the moisture of the diaper and that tender little behind.

Castor oil is a key ingredient here. Its thick, greasy texture is just right for protecting tiny bottoms from diaper rash. The gentle soothing properties in the Herbal Body Oil (page 26) add a little bit of moisturizing and conditioning, and natural wax helps bind everything together. Zinc oxide can be added to provide extra protection. The inclusion of zinc will give the ointment a thicker, more opaque quality while reinforcing baby's delicate skin and hopefully aiding in quick healing and recovery. Be sure to look for an uncoated, non-nano zinc oxide powder while shopping for ingredients. The powder should be advertised as having a particle size of at least 0.1 microns (100 nanometers). If the particle size is any smaller it may not be as effective and could potentially be a health concern.

INGREDIENTS

- 1 tablespoon and 1 teaspoon (35 ml) zinc oxide powder
- ½ cup (60 ml) Herbal Body Oil (recipe on page 26) or apricot kernel oil
- ¼ cup castor oil
- ½ cup (120 g) cocoa butter
- ½ cup (120 g) shea or mango butter
- 2 tablespoons (15 g) beeswax or candelilla wax

DIAPERING OINTMENTS *(continued)*

DIRECTIONS

1. Mix zinc oxide powder with 2 tablespoons Herbal Body Oil or apricot kernel oil in a small bowl; whisk until the ingredients are well blended. Set aside.

2. Combine the castor oil, the butters, remaining oil, and wax in a double boiler or a slow cooker set to low heat. Heat until the ingredients are fully melted.

3. Remove the mixture from the heat and let it sit for a few moments before carefully pouring about half of the mixture into one heatproof jar.

4. Mix the reserved oil and zinc mixture with the remaining melted oil and butter mixture. Allow the butter to cool to room temperature, whisking occasionally to disperse the zinc. When it has cooled to the touch and thickened to about the consistency of yogurt, it may be poured into a jar.

5. Allow both jars to cool and harden completely (about 2 hours) before use.

TO USE

I like to keep two jars of diapering ointment on hand: one with zinc and one without. I usually opt for the zinc ointment if my child already has a rash. For everyday care, I usually choose the zinc-free ointment.

ALL-OVER BABY WASH

Yield: 10 ounces (300 ml)

When it comes to life's greatest pleasures, the feeling of a freshly washed, wet little baby head against my cheek is right at the top. And holding that warm little bundle in a baby-sized terrycloth towel comes in at a very close second. While bath time isn't without its challenges, there's just something wonderful about a squeaky-clean baby—even if it only lasts a couple of minutes!

You can imagine why it puzzles me to find something as simple and pure as baby wash to be filled with impossible-to-pronounce and potentially toxic ingredients. Baby doesn't need all that yucky stuff. Really, you often don't need much more than water to keep your little one fresh and clean. On the occasions when a little extra is needed, I stick to a simple formula of liquid castile soap and herbal tea. This diluted liquid soap can be squirted onto a washcloth or pumped from a foaming dispenser to make scrubbing and shampooing even easier. Short on time? Just omit the herbs and use diluted liquid castile soap alone instead. After all, baby smells sweet enough as-is.

INGREDIENTS

- 1 cup (240 ml) water
- 2 tablespoons (4 g) dried lavender buds
- 2 tablespoons (4 g) dried chamomile
- ¼ cup (4 g) dried calendula
- ⅓ cup (80 ml) liquid castile soap

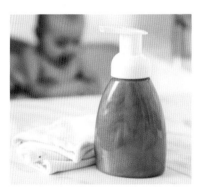

DIRECTIONS

1. Bring water to a boil.
2. Combine the boiled water with the lavender buds, chamomile, and calendula. Allow the herbs to steep in the water for about 30 minutes.
3. Strain the herbs from the water, then mix the water in with the castile soap.
4. Pour the mixture into a 10-ounce squirt bottle or foaming soap dispenser bottle.

TO USE

Squirt the soap liberally onto a washcloth or sponge, then work into a lather. Massage the lather gently onto baby's skin and hair before rinsing with water. Be careful to avoid getting soap into baby's eyes or mouth. This gentle soap is non-toxic, but it can be irritating if too much gets into the eyes. The diluted soap can be stored at room temperature for about 1 month or in the refrigerator for up to 3 months.

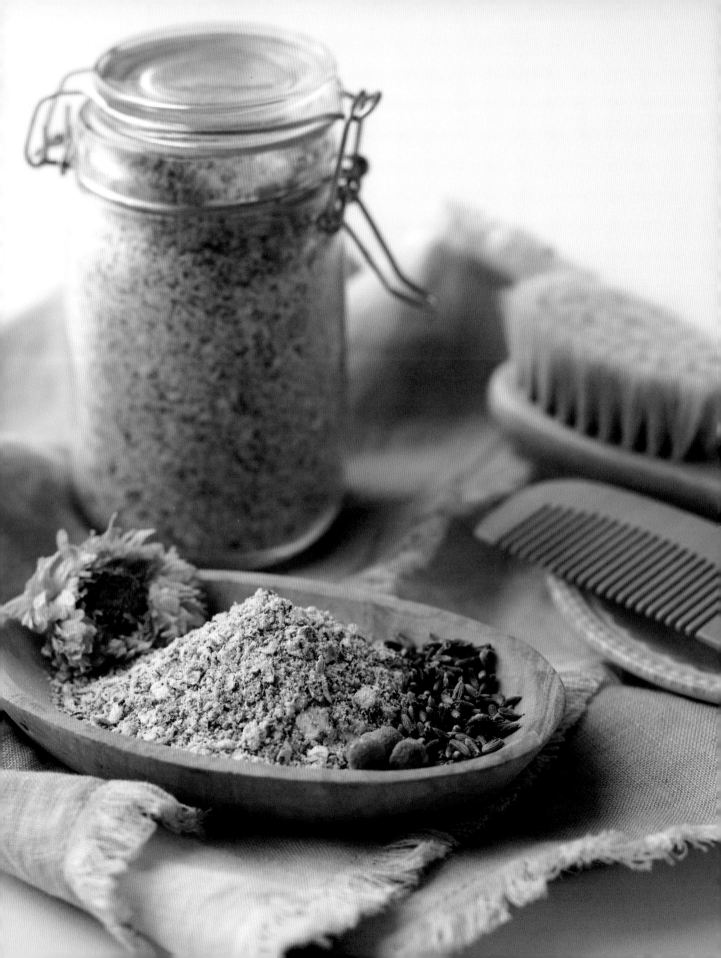

OATMEAL SCRUB

Yield: About 1/2 cup (120 ml)

was thrilled when my little one was born with a gorgeous head full of hair. His tiny furry head was as soft as silk and undeniably precious, but it wasn't too long before I started to see his scalp flake and crust. My poor baby! What was going on here?

Cradle cap is a very common for babies and toddlers, and while it may look pretty gnarly, it is usually nothing to worry about. Often, the symptoms of cradle cap can be tamed by giving baby a good shampoo and gentle scalp massage. If the cradle cap is especially stubborn, you might want to try giving your wee one a little home spa treatment using some moisturizing oil and a simple oatmeal scrub.

This recipe can also be used as a body scrub to help smooth minor bumps and scaliness from mild eczema or dryness.

If baby's skin or scalp seems unusually warm, or if the rash appears very red, or is cracked or oozing, see your doctor right away. In rare cases, cradle cap can require medication and treatment.

INGREDIENTS

- ¼ cup (60 ml) whole oats*
- ¼ cup (4 g) dried calendula
- 2 tablespoons (4 g) dried chamomile
- 2 tablespoons (4 g) dried lavender
- 1 cup hot water

*Use certified gluten-free oats if gluten allergies are a concern.

DIRECTIONS

1. Combine the oats and herbs in a food processor or blender and pulse until the mixture forms a uniform powder.

2. Transfer the mixture to a small muslin bag.

TO USE

Start off by applying a liberal amount of Herbal Body Oil (recipe on page 26) or plain apricot kernel oil to your baby's skin or scalp. Massage the oil onto baby very gently and allow it to soak in for at least 10 minutes before drawing a warm bath. Meanwhile, set the bag of herbs and oats in 1 cup of hot water and let it steep. Give baby a quick wash or shampoo, then remove the mixture from the bag and use it to gently scrub the affected area. Be sure not to use too much pressure; baby's hair is quite delicate and can be rubbed right off if you aren't careful! Follow the scrub with a rinse and a second wash or shampoo, if needed. Remove any flakes from baby's hair using a fine-tooth comb. If baby's skin or scalp feels dry after you've finished, rub in a few more drops of Herbal Body Oil as a moisturizer.

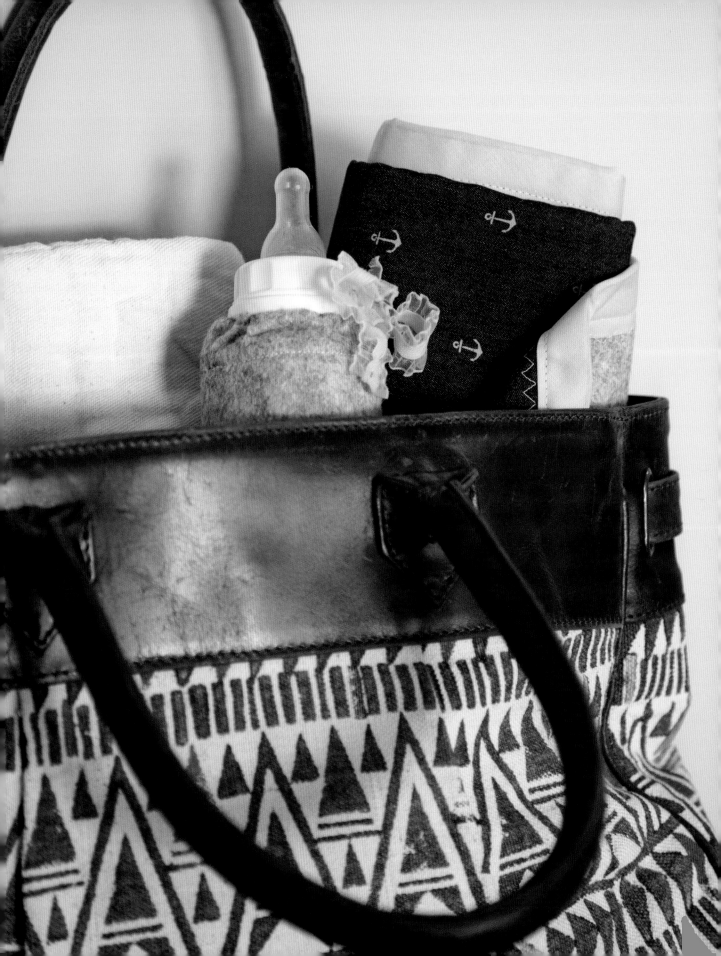

CHANGING MAT

Yield: 1 changing mat

I was never a big fan of the stiff and bulky changing mats that usually come with diaper bags. They tend to be a little too small for my wriggling child to lay on, but far too cumbersome to fit neatly in my bag. This simple fabric changing mat can be rolled into an efficiently sized bundle, but is large enough to let baby stretch out arms and legs comfortably while being changed.

If you find that this mat is still too large (or too small) for your liking, you can customize the project simply by adjusting the measurements to suit your own needs. I used a combination of soft comfy denim and moisture-blocking wool felt, but if you'd like something even more water resistant, try adding a layer of waterproof PUL to the bottom.

MATERIALS + TOOLS

- ½ (46cm) yard denim or canvas
- ½ (46cm) yard wool felt
- 1 3-yard (2.75m) package extra-wide double-fold bias tape
- Matching thread
- Scissors or a rotary cutter with mat
- Pins
- Ruler or measuring tape
- Cereal bowl or other round object
- Sewing machine

DIRECTIONS

Measure and Cut Pattern Pieces

1. Trim selvage edge from fabric. Measure and cut an 18 x 30-inch (46 x 76cm) rectangle from both the denim and wool felt.

2. Place the denim on top of the wool felt, right side up.

3. Use a cereal bowl or other round object to trace round quarter-circles on each corner. Cut round edges off rectangles, using traced shape (see figure 1, page 106).

Assemble Mat

4. Fold and pin the bias tape around the edges of the mat, being careful to line up both sides of the tape evenly. Sew the bias tape onto the mat by stitching close to its top edge (see figure 2, page 106).

5. Turn the mat over and check to see if both sides have been properly stitched. If any sections are still loose, stitch over them again.

CHANGING MAT *(continued)*

TO USE

Roll or fold up mat to fit easily into a diaper bag or backpack. Unroll when it's time to change and lay baby on the soft denim or canvas side of the mat. Launder as needed in hot water with baby-safe detergent. Air dry.

Figure 1

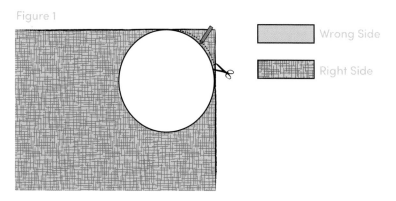

| | Wrong Side |
| | Right Side |

Figure 2

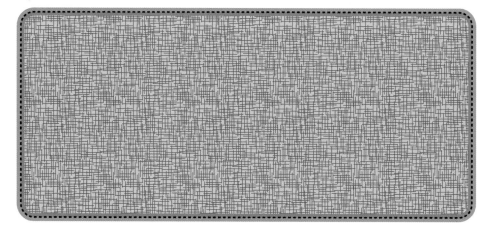

WASHCLOTH HAND PUPPET

Yield: 2 washcloth hand puppets

Whether bath time is your babe's favorite activity or most dreaded time of day, swapping out your regular washcloth for an adorable terrycloth hand puppet is sure to jazz things up. I left this pattern open to your imagination by giving the puppet a simple shape and a few interchangeable options for adding detail.

Both sets of ears can double as wings, arms, or flippers, allowing you to use the same pattern to make anything from a cute little chick to a baby beluga. Have fun with it! You can create your own creature or use the finished projects shown here as inspiration.

MATERIALS + TOOLS

- ½ yard (46cm) terrycloth
- Craft felt, various colors
- Matching thread
- Tracing paper and pencil
- Scissors or a rotary cutter with mat
- Pins
- Rulers or measuring tape
- Sewing machine

DIRECTIONS

Measure and Cut Pattern Pieces

1. Cut or trace pattern pieces (Washcloth Puppet A, Washcloth Puppet B, Washcloth Puppet C, Washcloth Puppet Embellishments) from pattern library (page 192).

2. Fold terrycloth in half. Pin pattern piece A to fabric with the arrow pointing toward the fold. Cut fabric, then repeat three more times to make four pieces.

3. Pin pattern piece B and C to folded fabric. Cut fabric and repeat to create four pieces from each pattern piece.

Make Ears/Eyes/Wings

4. Match up pairs of B pattern pieces with right sides in. Pin and sew around edges, leaving the bottom open to be turned out.

5. Match up pairs of C pattern pieces with right sides in. Pin and sew around edges, leaving the bottom open to be turned out.

6. Turn out B and C pieces (see page 20).

WASHCLOTH HAND PUPPET *(continued)*

Assemble Puppets

7. Match both pairs of the Washcloth Puppet A pattern piece together and pin edges. Place finished B or C pieces on between A pieces at spots indicated by X on the pattern. You may use the spots on top to give the puppets ears or eyes, or use the spots on the side to give the puppet wings, fins, or arms.

8. Sew around edges of each pair using a ⅛-inch (3mm) seam allowance, leaving the bottom of the puppet open for turning out (see figure 1, page 109).

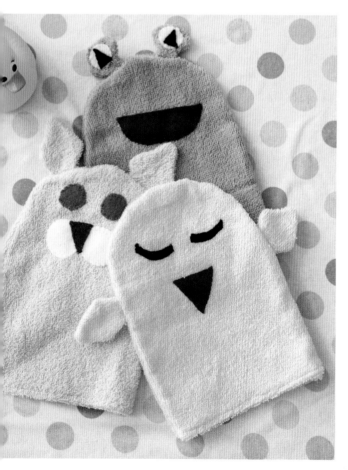

9. Go over the edges that you've just sewn with a narrow zigzag stitch. This extra step will help stop the fabric from fraying and extend the life of your puppet.

Hem Puppets

10. Fold the bottom of each finished piece up by ½ inch (13mm) and fold it once more by an additional ½ inch (13mm), pin the folded fabric down, and sew around hem (see figure 2, page 109).

Finish Puppets

11. Turn out puppet. Use embellishment patterns to cut face shapes from craft felt. Try using the circle for eyes, cheeks, or a surprised mouth. Try using the triangle for ears, eyes, or a beak. The curved shape can be used to make a smile.

12. Hand-stitch embellishments onto the finished puppets using needle and thread (instructions on page 19; see figure 3, page 109).

TO USE

Wear your washcloth hand puppets to put on a show at tubby time, and to gently scrub your little one with soapy bubbles. Wash on gentle cycle with cold water. Air dry.

WASHCLOTH HAND PUPPET (continued)

Figure 1

Right Side

Wrong Side

Felt

Figure 2

Figure 3

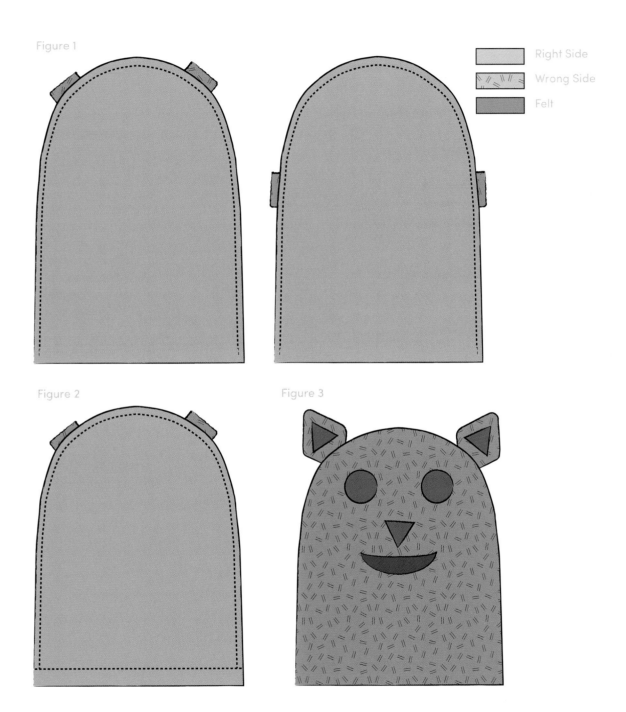

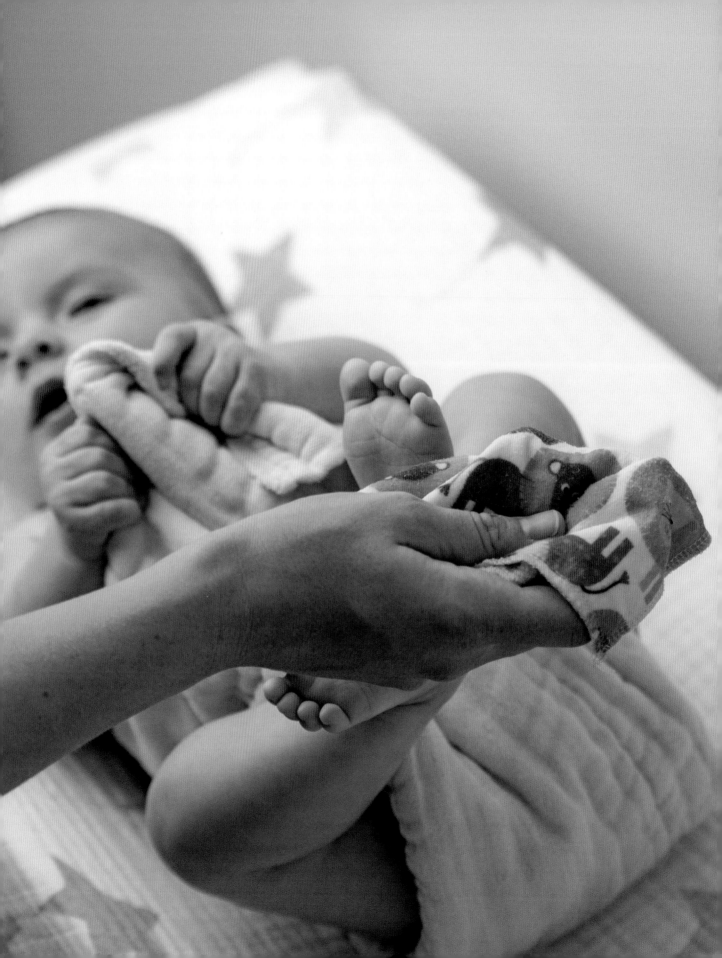

CLOTH BABY WIPES

Yield: Makes about 24 baby wipes

There are few parenting tasks less glamorous than wiping a dirty bum. It's a thankless, stinky job, but as many a mama has said before me, "Ya do whatcha gotta do." There is, however, one way to make bum-wiping a *little* more enjoyable, and that's by doing the job with all-natural, totally reusable, and optionally adorable cloth baby wipes.

Not only are cloth baby wipes much prettier than disposable wipes, they can save mom and dad a bundle of cash and help reduce baby's environmental footprint. Just think—a typical infant goes through anywhere from five to ten diaper changes per day, and each change might use one to three wipes. That means you could go through *thousands* of wipes in the first three months alone—and baby could be rocking diapers for years! Building a stash of cloth baby wipes is a relatively easy way to increase the economic and ecological sustainability of the whole endeavor.

Prep your fabric before starting this project by washing it in hot water with diaper-safe detergent and without any fabric softener. Dry the fabric on a normal cycle, but don't use any fabric softener or dryer sheets here either. Softeners and dryer sheets can build up a residue on the wipes that will make them less absorbent. Use these same washing instructions to launder your wipes once you start using them.

MATERIALS + TOOLS

- 1 yard (91cm) flannel
- 1 yard (91cm) terrycloth
- Matching thread
- Scissors or a rotary cutter with mat
- Pins
- Ruler or measuring tape
- Sewing machine or serger (for finishing)

DIRECTIONS

Measure and Cut Pattern Pieces

1. Measure and cut 24 8-inch (20cm) squares from the terrycloth and the flannel fabric.

Assemble Wipes

2. Place one square of flannel on top of one square of terrycloth. If either fabric has a pattern or texture, make sure to place the wrong sides in and the right sides out—just like you'd like the finished product to look (see figure 1, page 112).

3. If you are using a sewing machine, set it to a tight zigzag stitch, then sew around the entire outer edge of the fabric squares as close to the edge as you can manage. Be sure to backstitch at the beginning and end to secure your stitching (see figure 2, right).

4. If you are using a serger, simply run the serger over the outer edge of the fabric to finish it.

Finish Wipes

5. Use a pair of scissors to snip off any dangling pieces of fabric or thread, and to trim off any excess fabric around the edges. Be careful not to snip any of the stitching as you trim.

Finish Batch

6. Repeat with the remaining squares of fabric.

TO USE

The wipes should be soaked with plain water just before use, or they can be stored soaking wet in an electric wipe warmer. If you decide to use a wipe warmer, make sure that it is cleaned and disinfected every day. The wetted wipes should also be replaced once every day to prevent any bacteria from building up.

Figure 1

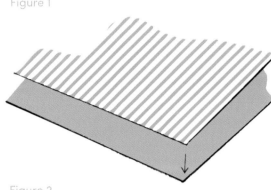

Figure 2

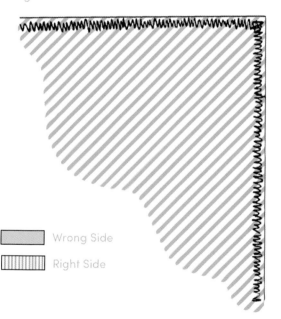

Wrong Side

Right Side

UPCYCLED T-SHIRT TOUK

YIELD: *1 baby hat*

Is there anything more comfy or nostalgic than a favorite T-shirt? This project gives your tattered old T-shirts a second life as a cozy and customized hat for baby. Pay homage to your favorite rock band, a memorable vacation, or even your old alma mater.

I used a T-shirt from a favorite local farm for this project. If you don't have any T-shirts handy, knit jersey can be purchased by the yard from most fabric stores. It's sometimes available in cute prints too. You can even get extra artistic and try your hand at embellishing a plain T-shirt or piece of jersey with fabric paint, silk screening, or iron-on transfers.

MATERIALS + TOOLS

- 1 adult-sized T-shirt
- Matching thread
- Tracing paper and pencil
- Scissors or a rotary cutter with mat
- Pins
- Ruler or measuring tape
- Sewing machine

DIRECTIONS

Measure and Cut Pattern Pieces

1. Cut or trace pattern pieces (T-Shirt Touk A) from pattern library (page 191).

2. Lay the T-shirt flat, then place the pattern piece over the section you would like to feature on the hat. Make sure the section of T-shirt you are using stretches horizontally (see figure 1, page 115).

3. Pin the pattern piece down and cut.

Assemble Hat

4. Place two right sides of fabric together and pin. Stitch all around sides and top of hat, leaving the bottom edge open for turning out (see figure 2, page 115).

Hem Hat

5. Turn out fabric, then fold bottom up by ½ inch (13mm) and then again by an additional 1/2 inch (13mm). Pin to secure.

6. Turn hat sideways and stitch vertically up the folded hem on both sides of the hat (see figure 3, page 115).

Finish Hat

7. Tie the hat's long top tip in a small knot (see figure 4, page 115).

TO USE

Pop on baby's head any time. Wash on gentle cycle with cold water. Dry on low heat.

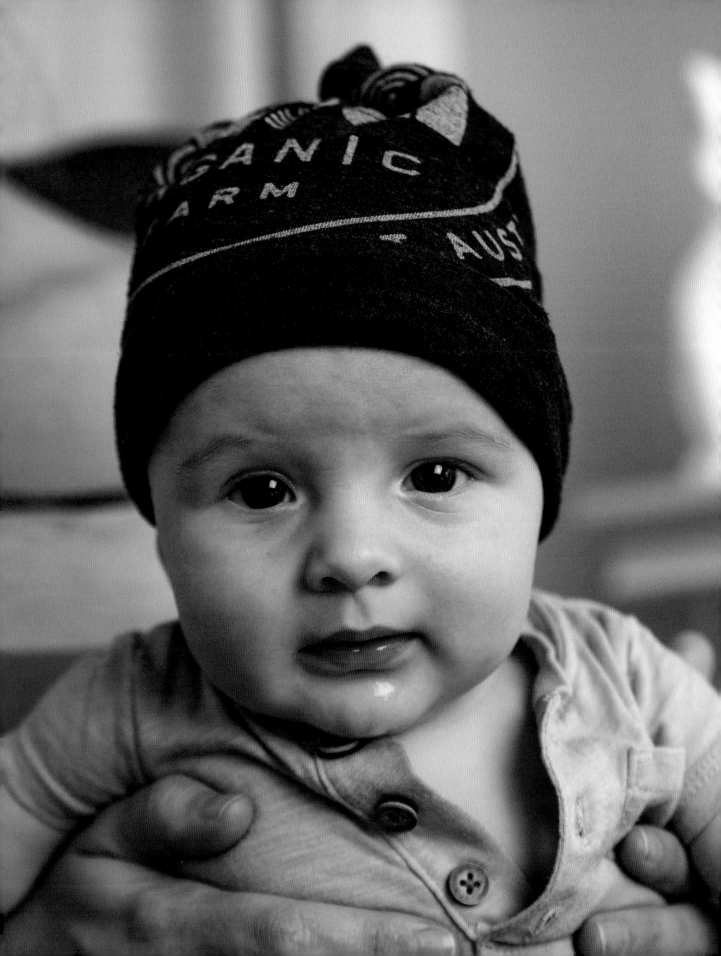

UPCYCLED T-SHIRT TOUK (continued)

Figure 1

Figure 2

Wrong Side

Right Side

Pattern

Fabric Stretch

Figure 3

Figure 4

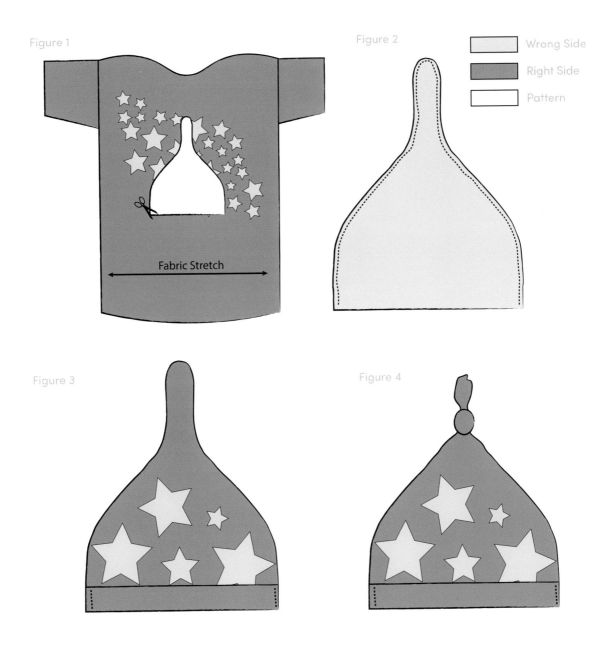

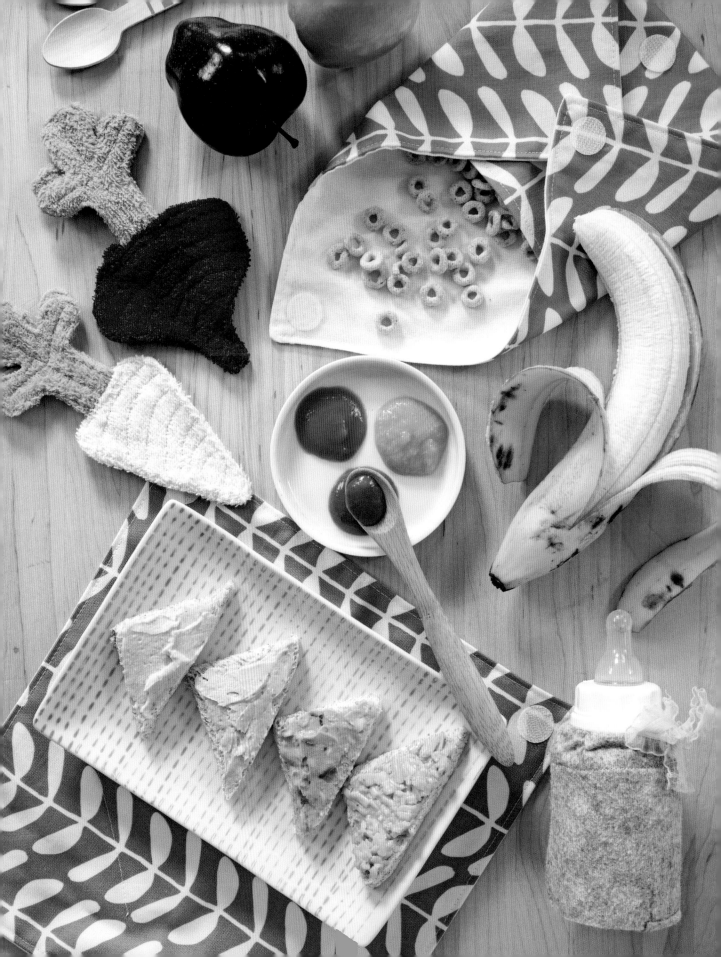

↓

chapter 4

FEEDING BABY

Ahh, breast-feeding—one of the signature features of our mammalian heritage. We carry our babies until they reach the right stage of development, then out they come, ready to suckle from our shapely bosom, which is, of course, just bursting with milk.

Sounds easy, right? I discovered, like just about every other mother on earth, that nursing your baby can be a lot more challenging than expected—and that it's just the beginning of a long journey of nourishing your child and teaching them to nourish themselves. Whether you are nursing, pumping, bottle-feeding, using formula, or working with a combination of these methods, all of us mamas have a common goal: feeding our babies!

While the medical community can prove which method is best for baby's health and development from a scientific standpoint, it can't determine which choice will be right for you as an individual or what actually works well for your family. To tell you the truth, you may not be able to determine that either until you are in the thick of it, making difficult choices in an effort to keep yourself and your family healthy, happy, and well fed.

Wherever your baby's food journey takes you, it is sure to be a wild ride! Get ready for your life to become a lot stickier, but also a lot more fun. Even if you don't find food-covered babies to be particularly adorable now, just wait until it's *your* baby coated in pumpkin puree. That's some pretty heart-melting stuff right there—at least I think so. ➡

starting solid foods

Most pediatricians recommend keeping baby on a strict diet of only breastmilk or formula until somewhere in the range of four to six months. Lately, more and more pediatricians are leaning toward the later end of that window or even giving the opinion that babies should always wait until they reach six months before trying solid foods. Like so many aspects of childcare, it doesn't seem to be an exact science. If you aren't sure whether your child is ready or not, talk to your pediatrician.

When baby is finally ready to get started with new foods, you'll have some choices to make. Which foods will you try first? Will you give baby purees or try out baby-led weaning, a method that allows babies to gnaw on whole foods instead of being spoon-fed? Will you make your own organic food at home or take advantage of the ready-made jars in the baby food aisle? The whole thing can seem surprisingly overwhelming!

The truth is that you can turn almost any kind of food into baby puree simply by throwing it into the blender with a little water or breastmilk. Rocket science, this is not. However, there are a few things you do need to keep in mind while cooking for baby:

ALLERGIES AND SENSITIVITIES

Allergic reactions can be really scary— sometimes even deadly. That's one reason most pediatricians recommend introducing foods to babies slowly and methodically during the first few months. Make sure to keep track of how your child reacts to each new food, especially with the most common allergens such as nuts, dairy, eggs, gluten, shellfish, and soy. If your child has any family history of serious allergies, make sure to talk to the doctor before introducing these foods.

SALT

Babies under one year old cannot tolerate more than 1 gram of salt per day. Their little kidneys are just not well-developed enough to handle the level of salt that most adults consume. For this reason, I choose to omit salt from my homemade baby food all-together. This is also a really important thing to keep in mind when sharing your own meals with baby.

SWEETENERS

While honey makes an excellent natural sweetener later in life, babies should not be given honey (or foods that contain honey) until they are at least one year old. Honey can contain botulism spores that tiny bodies are not equipped to deal with. This can lead to botulism poisoning, a potentially deadly condition. Maple syrup, corn syrup, and other sweetening syrups are not as commonly associated with botulism poisoning but they still pose the same risk, and should be kept off limits until your baby reaches that first birthday. Artificial sweeteners pose a whole other variety of possible health risks, so

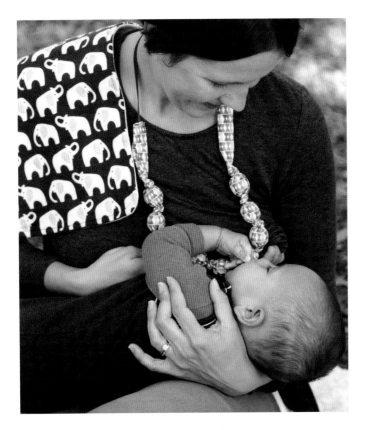

Baby may not like something the first time it is tried, but that doesn't mean it will be despised forever. In fact, babies sometimes need to try new flavors or textures repeatedly before giving them a real shot.

fad diets aren't for babies

The people who know me best know that I love a good specialty diet. I grew up as an ovo-lacto-vegetarian, dabbled in veganism, and even went paleo for a while. I've survived several juice cleanses too. Of course, being an adult, I am free to experiment with, indulge, or even abuse my diet in any way I please. Babies, on the other hand, may have needs that exceed the limitations of a specialty diet, especially any kind of diet that purposely excludes certain types of nutrients like fat or carbs. That's not saying that you can't raise your child to be vegan or even gluten-free, but it's important to keep the baby's diverse nutritional needs in mind as you plan meals. Talking to your doctor about how your child's diet may differ or align with your own is a great way to make sure everyone in the family stays happy and healthy.

eating out with little ones

Venturing out of the house with a wee one in tow can sometimes be intimidating, especially around meal time. Kids don't generally care for being strapped in, told to quiet down, or made to sit still. They

are also best avoided. Sweeteners are rarely needed for feeding babies, but if sweetening a food or baked good is necessary, look to pureed fruits and good old-fashioned granulated sugar.

SHAPE AND TEXTURE

While introducing baby to new foods, try to keep their limitations in mind. Thick foods, like nut butters, must be thinned out considerably before being spoon-fed to an infant. Otherwise, the thick, sticky texture could become a choking hazard. When you introduce finger foods, make sure the food is served in manageable bites that are smaller in size than baby's windpipe.

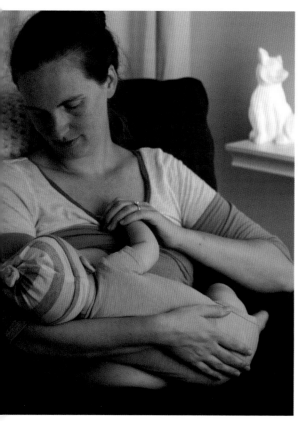

COME PREPARED

Baby might love everything you order and be as pleased as can be to share with Mom. But then again, maybe not. Make sure to pack baby-friendly foods and snacks. A toy or two wouldn't hurt either.

TAKE A WALK

Baby will probably not want to sit still through your entire meal. It can help to take a quick stroll between the time you order and when your food arrives. If you are dining with a friend, ask them to walk baby around again while you are waiting for the bill.

PLAN YOUR ESCAPE

Ask for to-go containers and the bill as early as you can. This will make you ready for a quick escape in the case of diaper explosions, temper tantrums, mommy meltdowns, or other such disasters.

BEND, DON'T BREAK

I've eaten dim sum with chopsticks while nursing my toddler in the middle of a packed restaurant. It wasn't our best dinner out, but it was Mother's Day, we were on vacation, and I intended to finish that meal come hell or high water. Sometimes you have to get creative in order to make it through an outing gone wrong. Sometimes you have to give up and eat at home instead. Either way, do your best to stay cool, be flexible, and accept that this is all part of the ride.

aren't particularly neat or orderly eaters either! The truth is that eating meals out with kids can be difficult, but like so many aspects of parenthood, just because it's hard doesn't mean you shouldn't do it anyway. In fact, I have a few tips that may help:

EMBRACE HAPPY HOUR

Restaurants are the quietest and most child-friendly between 3 and 5 p.m. As an added bonus, many restaurants offer food and drink specials at that time as well. The biggest advantage of eating before 5 p.m. is that kids' moods tend to be lighter while the sun is up. Win win win.

ASK AN *expert*

Q: **How can I tell if my baby is eating enough?**

A: The average baby will feed eight to twelve times a day and come off the breast "milk drunk" and content. Diaper output also tells us that baby is transferring (and digesting!) well.

Q: **Can the foods I eat affect my breastmilk?**

A: Rarely! The quality of your breastmilk is well-protected. That means if you are too busy to cook a healthy meal, or skip the occasional meal, your milk will still contain all the exact nutrients your baby needs. Eating perfectly is not necessary to make the perfect food for your baby. When you eat a wide variety of foods in as close to their natural state as possible, it will help give *you* the energy to mother your baby.

Q: **How can I tell if my baby is full or still hungry?**

A: If you have a baby who just loves staying on the breast forever, consider two things: your little one may enjoy the comfort of being close to you long after the tummy is full, or baby may be having trouble transferring milk effectively (and so tires quickly, takes a rest while still on the nipple, and then wakes and continues feeding). If you suspect the latter, you would benefit from calling the La Leche League helpline in your area, or an International Board-Certified Lactation Consultant (IBCLC).

—*Tanja Knutson, International Board-Certified Lactation Consultant (IBCLC), tanjaknutson.com*

nursing support

If you choose to breast-feed your baby, there are two things that are very important to keep in mind. The first thing to know is that breastfeeding isn't always easy. Most mothers face multiple challenges along the way. From milk production issues to tongue ties and plain old logistics, it can sometimes feel like your breast-feeding goals are far out of reach. That might sound a little scary, but there is one more thing to remember. Women have been nursing babies for a very long time, and while you may be brand new to the practice as an individual, we mamas have quite a bit of expertise as a community. No matter what challenge you and your baby are facing, if breast-feeding is important to you, there are people out there who want to help you find a solution.

LA LECHE LEAGUE

The La Leche League (LLL) has been helping breast-feeding mamas for more than sixty years. The organization hosts support groups, classes, and meetups all over the world and hosts an online forum. Find a leader near you at llli.org.

LOCAL SUPPORT GROUPS

Connecting with other moms and hearing about how they've overcome their own challenges can be both helpful and inspiring. Look for breast-feeding support groups on sites like meetup.com or kellymom.com.

LACTATION CONSULTANTS

An International Board-Certified Lactation Consultant (IBCLC) is a great choice for private one-on-one help. They usually do charge a fee for private consultation. It's worth checking with your health insurance provider to see whether you are covered for the service.

ONLINE COMMUNITIES AND FORUMS

If you prefer anonymity, or just can't manage to leave the house (been there), online forums can be helpful too. Just remember that while forums are a great place to share and connect with other mamas, they are no substitute for advice from an expert.

the first birthday

Baby's first birthday is a milestone you may never forget. Whether or not you decide to plan a party, I highly recommend planning some kind of indulgence or acknowledgement for you and your partner or spouse, or anyone else who may have been instrumental in making it through the past year. While every birthday after this one will undoubtedly revolve around your child,

ASK AN *expert*

Q: Do you have any tips to share on feeding babies and toddlers who are picky or unenthusiastic eaters?

A: Don't take it personally! Kids are allowed to have tastes. At the same time, we shape those tastes with exposure. If you continue to serve a healthy, well-rounded diet—and refuse to fight or engage in dinnertime drama when they go through periods where they want no part of it—you'll eventually raise healthy, well-rounded eaters.

—*Stacie Billis, food editor and cookbook author, eats.coolmompicks.com*

the first birthday is also a celebration for you, the caregivers. Treat yourself to something nice—even if that something nice is simply a well-deserved pat on the back or some special alone time to reminisce with a diary or photo album. This isn't just your child's birthday; it's the anniversary of the day you met your baby face to face, and that, mama, is a very big deal.

EASY BABY FOOD PUREES

Pureed baby food is probably the most popular and easily the most iconic way to introduce new foods to tiny babies. When you find out just how easy it is to make your own all-natural baby food, it might make you wonder how baby food manufacturers stay in business. I have a theory—those tiny multi-colored jars are too cute to resist!

Making your own purees at home is super simple though, especially if you invest in a few basic tools. Having a blender or food processor makes mushing up all that delicious food a total snap. The food mill, a simple hand-cranked device, even eliminates the need for peeling and seeding fruits. Add a small saucepan for boiling fruits, vegetables, and grains to your stash and you are good to go.

Another great thing to invest in is a set of high-quality silicone ice cube trays. These trays allow you to freeze individual portions of baby food. Just freeze the cubes and then pop them into tubs or baggies. Homemade baby food can be stored in the freezer for up to three months.

FAVORITE COMBINATIONS

- Peaches and sweet potato with cinnamon
- Berries, yogurt, and oatmeal
- Chicken and mashed potato
- Lentils and apples with cinnamon
- Apricots and raspberries with parsnips
- Spinach and blueberries with brown rice

DIRECTIONS

1. Prepare any combination (or just a single ingredient) according to the table on page 125. Add liquid as needed to achieve a thin texture similar to applesauce.

2. Allow the puree to cool before serving it to baby or spooning it into ice cube trays to be frozen.

3. To thaw, simply pop a cube of baby food into an airtight container and store in the fridge overnight. Or, you can speed up the process by heating the frozen puree in a small saucepan over low-medium heat. Cook until thoroughly heated and allow to cool to room temperature before feeding baby.

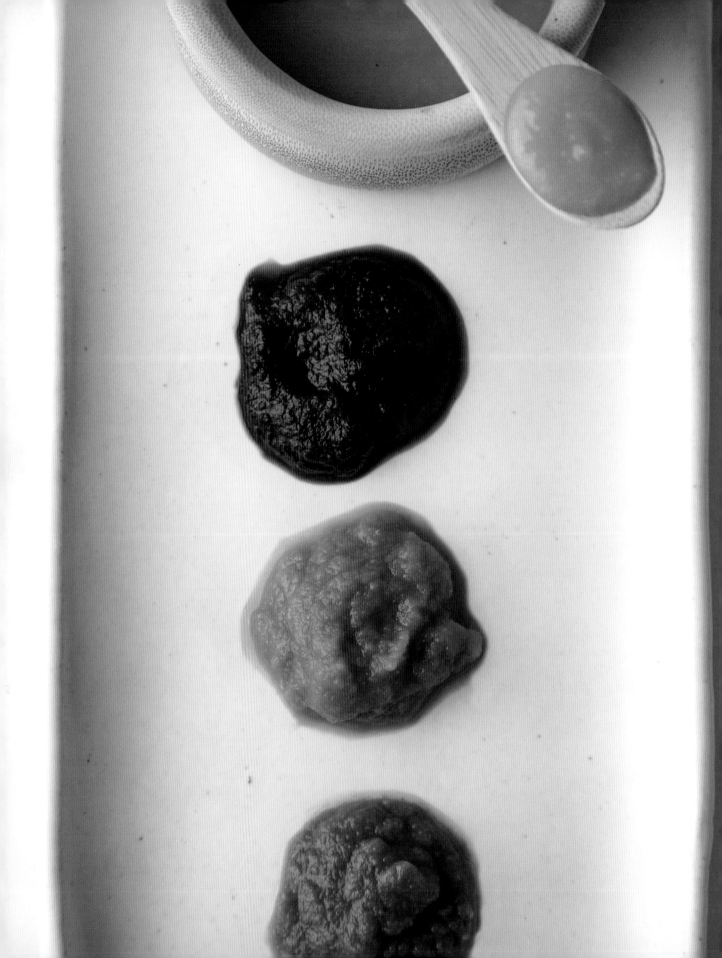

EASY BABY FOOD PUREES *(continued)*

PREPARATION OF VARIOUS FRUITS AND VEGETABLES

CATEGORY	INGREDIENT	PREPARATION
Stone Fruits	Apple, apricot, nectarine, peach, plum	Cut into quarters, remove pits, and boil until soft (about 20 to 30 minutes). Push through food mill to puree and remove skins, or peel and grate before cooking.
Soft Fruits and Berries	Blueberries, melon, raspberries, strawberries	Mash raw or puree with blender.
Grains and Beans	Oatmeal, barley, beans, brown rice, lentils, quinoa, white rice	Cook to soften, then puree in blender with liquid until smooth.
Meat, Fish, and Poultry	Chicken, ground beef, salmon	Poach in boiling water until cooked through (15 to 20 minutes). Remove skin and bones. Puree in blender with liquid.
Starchy Vegetables	Parsnips, potato, sweet potato	Peel and quarter, boil until very soft (about 20 to 30 minutes), and mash with fork.
Other Vegetables	Asparagus, carrots, green beans, peas, kale, spinach	Boil until soft and then puree in blender until smooth.
Liquids	Breastmilk, homemade or sodium-free broth, formula, plain yogurt, water	Use to wet ingredients for purees.
Spices	Basil, cinnamon, coriander, cumin, curry, dill, garlic, ginger	Include a pinch in baby food purees to add interesting flavors.

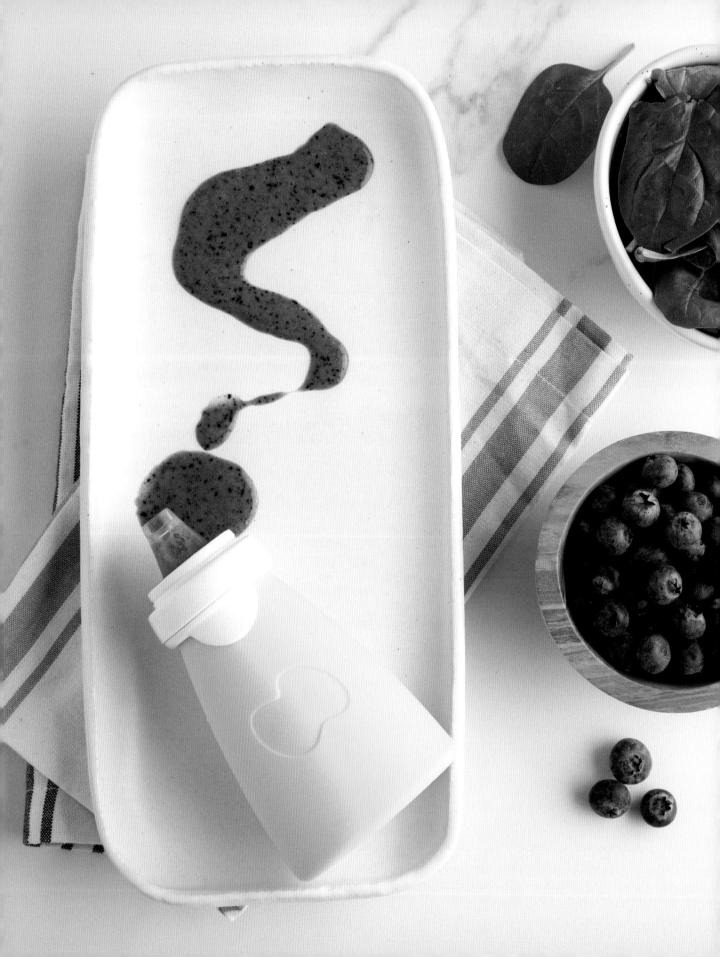

SQUEEZY POUCH SMOOTHIES

YIELD: *About 2 4-ounce (120 ml) servings each*

Smoothies are a quick and easy way to keep little ones happily hydrated while filling them up with nutritious fruits and veggies. The following recipes have a thinner consistency and a lower amount of sugar than recipes typically made for adults. They are still a bit too chunky to fit through a sippy cup, but reusable squeeze pouches are an excellent delivery method. Babykins will love squishing that business right up into his cute little face. In the height of his squeezy pouch obsession, my son could empty an entire pouch in no more than 30 seconds.

Find reusable pouches with other children's kitchenware in grocery stores, children's boutiques, or online. When shopping for smoothie ingredients, choose organic fruits and vegetables whenever possible. This is especially important when it comes to soft fruits like berries, as they are usually treated with a higher dose of pesticides than other kinds of produce. Look for organic full-fat or whole milk yogurts in either plain or vanilla flavors. Steer clear of any yogurts that are non-fat or include honey or artificial flavors and added sweeteners.

DIRECTIONS

1. Place any liquid ingredients into the bottom of the blender first, followed by the fresh ingredients. Place the frozen ingredients into the blender last.

2. Secure the top of the blender, then blend at a slow speed for 30 seconds. Increase to a high speed and blend for 2 minutes.

3. If the smoothie ends up being too thick or chunky to blend easily, try adding 1 or 2 tablespoons of water or breastmilk and blending again.

4. If the mixture is at all fibrous or chunky, pour through a fine mesh strainer before transferring into squeeze pouch. Pouches can be served right away or refrigerated for up to 3 days or frozen for up to 3 months.

INGREDIENTS

Blueberry-Spinach Smoothie

- ½ banana
- ½ cup (120 ml) frozen blueberries
- ¼ cup (60 ml) baby spinach
- ¼ cup (60 ml) water or breastmilk
- ¼ cup (60 ml) plain whole milk yogurt

Mango-Carrot Smoothie

- ½ banana
- ½ cup (120 ml) frozen mango
- ¼ cup (60 ml) frozen carrots
- ¼ cup (60 ml) water or breastmilk
- ¼ cup (60 ml) plain whole milk yogurt

Berry Bell Smoothie

- ½ banana
- ½ cup (120 ml) frozen strawberries
- ¼ cup (60 ml) diced red bell peppers
- ¼ cup (60 ml) water or breastmilk
- ¼ cup (60 ml) plain whole milk yogurt

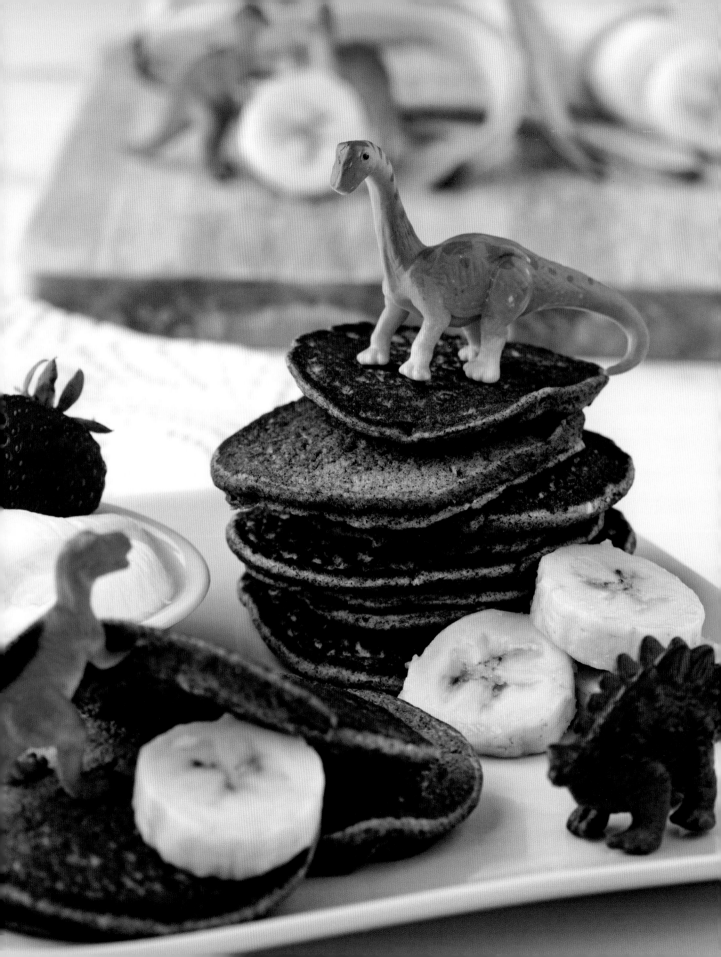

HILAH'S BANANA PANCAKES

YIELD: *About 24 mini pancakes*

This recipe comes from my dear friend and fellow mama, Hilah Johnson of Hilah Cooking (hilahcooking.com). Hilah and I became mommies within just a handful of months of each other and I was grateful to have another lady in my life who approached the whole endeavor with a similar sense of humor. We joked about making mistakes. We shared our fears and our triumphs. We watched in horror as my baby poked hers in the eye. Hilah was a huge part of my own beginnings as a mother, so I couldn't imagine writing this book without some of her input. When I asked her to share a recipe for baby, she suggested banana pancakes. The following recipe and introduction are from Hilah:

It is *hard* to find good toddler recipes, meaning things that can be made ahead and reheated; things that aren't complicated; things that my toddler will actually eat. Made without egg, the pancakes are thinner and a little more delicate; made with egg, they are thicker and puffier and fairly sturdy.

So besides the fact that these banana pancakes can be made with or without eggs, the other marvelous thing about making pancakes for toddlers is they hold up great in the fridge for a week. Cook, cool, then layer between waxed paper and store covered. Reheat in the toaster for a quick breakfast. You definitely want to layer some waxed paper between them because they will stick together otherwise and ruin your morning. If you want to freeze them, you can do that, too! Again, single layer of pancakes on waxed paper or parchment, freeze solid, then store in freezer bags or boxes. Thaw as needed.

INGREDIENTS

- 1 ripe banana or ½ cup sweet potato, boiled and mashed
- 1 egg or 1 tablespoon (15 ml) oil
- 1¼ cups (300 ml) milk or non-dairy milk
- ½ teaspoon (2.5 ml) vanilla extract, optional
- Dash cinnamon, optional
- ¾ cup (180 ml) whole wheat flour or all-purpose gluten-free flour (page 30)
- ½ cup (120 ml) buckwheat flour
- 1 teaspoon (5 ml) baking powder
- Oil for cooking (I like coconut oil)

HILAH'S BANANA PANCAKES *(continued)*

DIRECTIONS

1. Mash banana in a large bowl with a fork until it's mostly smooth; substitute boiled and mashed sweet potato if you prefer the pancakes to be less sweet. Mix in egg (if using). Add milk, oil (if using), and vanilla and stir well.

2. Add dry ingredients and mix quickly. There may be some lumps.

3. Lightly oil a griddle and heat over medium. It is ready when a drop of water will sizzle on it.

4. Portion batter by large tablespoonfuls, spreading the batter out to make a circle about 2 inches (5cm) in diameter. Cook until the edges begin to look dry and bubbles form around the outside. Use a spatula to flip each pancake and cook another 1 to 2 minutes until brown and crispy.

5. Serve pancakes hot with butter and syrup, or cool to refrigerate or freeze. Pancakes can be reheated in a toaster or toaster oven.

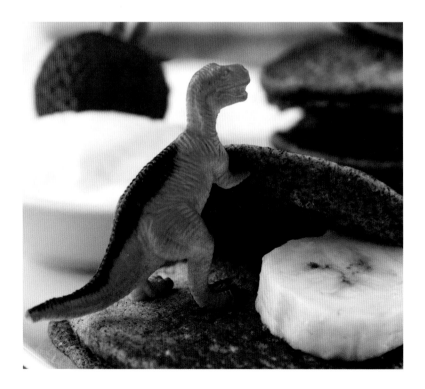

SLOW-COOKED APPLE BUTTER

YIELD: *6 ounces (175 ml)*

Have you ever wished you could smush up an apple and smear it on a piece of toast? Then this is your lucky day. Apple butter is basically a concentrated apple jam that cooks down, low and slow, until it reaches a thick, smooth consistency that spreads like, well, butter.

My slow-cooked apple butter is made without any additional sugar, yielding the nice mellow apple flavor that babies like best. This spread is perfect for making sandwiches, flavoring yogurt or oatmeal, or as a dip for pancakes. If your babe has an adventurous palate, try adding a dash of cinnamon to this recipe for extra flavor.

As a mama, I've really grown to love recipes that basically cook themselves. Apple butter definitely qualifies. This simple fruit spread takes several hours to cook, but once the initial work of peeling and chopping is over, the butter can be left to simmer away unattended. The apples will disintegrate as they cook, making pureeing totally unnecessary.

I prefer to make my apple butter in a slow cooker so I don't have to worry about leaving my stove on all day. If you don't have a slow cooker, that's okay. A regular pot on the stovetop will do. Just keep the burner turned to low and check in on its progress, and maybe give it a stir a little more often.

You can use any variety of apple for this recipe. The butter's flavor will vary depending on the variety of apple you pick. A butter made with Honeycrisp apples will be sweeter, while a butter made with Granny Smith apples will be more tart. By the way, this method can also be used to make peach, nectarine, or apricot butter. Just remove the peels and pits before cooking and you are good to go!

INGREDIENTS

- 2 pounds (0.9 kg) apples (about 5 apples)
- 2 cups (480 ml) water
- 2 tablespoons (30 ml) lemon juice
- ¼ teaspoon cinnamon (optional)

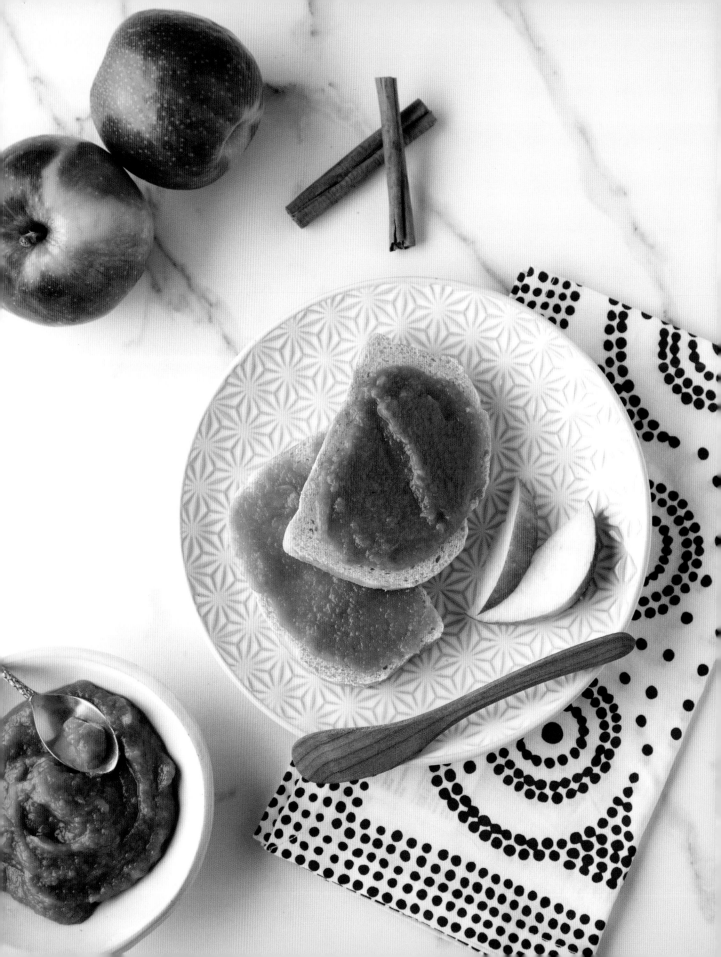

SLOW-COOKED APPLE BUTTER *(continued)*

DIRECTIONS

1. Peel apples and cut into quarters, removing and discarding core.

2. Place apples in pot or slow cooker along with water, lemon juice, and cinnamon (if using).

3. If using slow cooker, cover and cook on high for 1 hour, then on low for 8 hours, stirring occasionally. If using stove top, cover and bring to a boil, then reduce to low heat and simmer for 4 to 6 hours, stirring occasionally.

4. When the apples have disintegrated and the butter has become very thick and deep brown in color, remove from heat and allow to cool to room temperature. Cooled apple butter may be stored in the refrigerator for up to 2 weeks or in the freezer for up to 3 months.

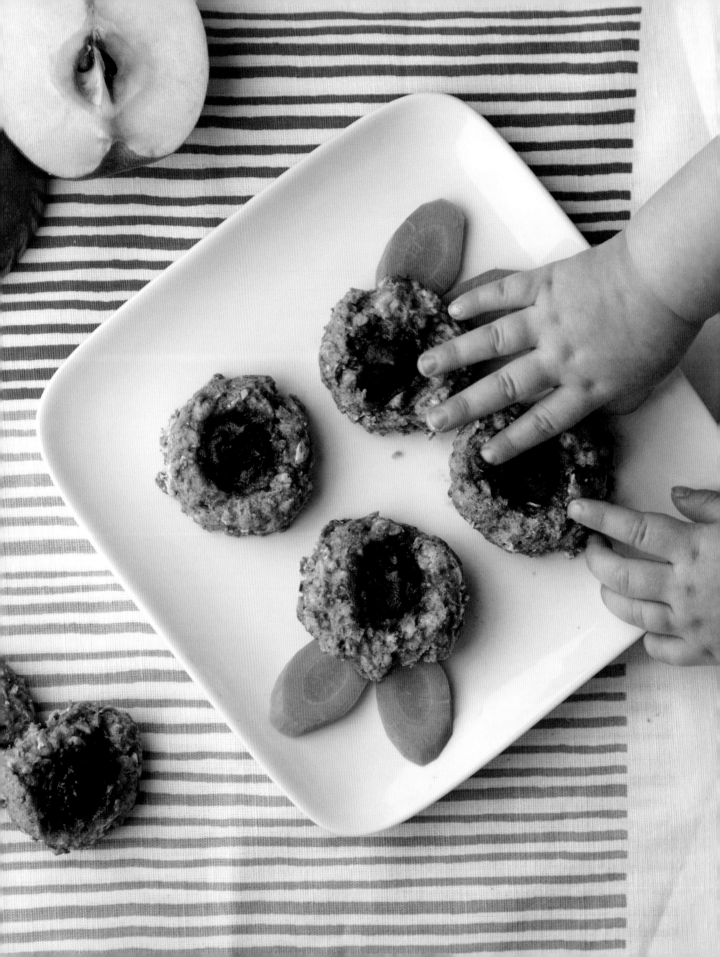

OATMEAL CARROT THUMBPRINT COOKIES

YIELD: *About 12 cookies*

After my son started eating solid food it wasn't too long before he became fixated on one food over another. One such obsession (which still persists even at two years old) was for pre-packaged fruit bars. There are a great many brands out there to choose from—some more healthy than others—but nothing beats making your own at home.

Of course, making nutritious layered cookies filled with fruit puree is a bit too labor intensive for busy mamas like myself. I invented these simple thumbprint cookies as a sort of cheater version of the illustrious fruit bar. They are packed with healthy ingredients (I even sneak carrots into these) and topped with a dollop of homemade apple butter. The kids? They go gaga.

INGREDIENTS

- 1 cup (240 ml) quick-cooking oats
- 1 cup (240 ml) whole wheat flour or all-purpose gluten free flour (recipe page 30)
- ½ teaspoon (2.5 ml) baking powder
- 1 teaspoon (5 ml) cinnamon
- ½ cup (120 ml) raw carrots, minced or shredded
- ¾ (180 ml) cup sugar
- ¼ cup (60 ml) almond or sunflower butter
- 1 tablespoon (15 ml) coconut oil or melted butter
- 1 egg or 2 tablespoons (30 ml) applesauce
- ¼ cup (60 ml) slow-cooked apple butter (recipe page 131)

DIRECTIONS

1. Preheat oven to 350°F (177°C). Line two baking sheets with parchment or silicone liners.

2. Whisk together oats, flour, baking powder, and cinnamon in a large bowl and set aside.

3. In the bowl of a stand mixer fitted with a beater attachment, combine carrots, sugar, almond or sunflower butter, coconut oil or melted butter, and egg or applesauce. Beat until well blended.

4. Slowly stir the dry ingredients into the wet and mix until just combined.

5. Form balls of dough using about 2 tablespoons each, and line them up on the baking sheets. Use your finger (or thumb) to form a shallow depression in each cookie, flattening them slightly.

OATMEAL CARROT THUMBPRINT COOKIES *(continued)*

6. Fill each depression with about ½ teaspoon apple butter.

7. Bake for 12 to 15 minutes, turning the cookies halfway through baking time. If using gluten-free flour, bake for an extra 5 to 10 minutes, or until the cookies appear firm and slightly browned.

8. Allow the cookies to sit for about 10 minutes before removing them to cooling racks. Cookies may be enjoyed as soon as they are cool enough to eat. They can be refrigerated for up to 1 week or frozen for up to 6 months.

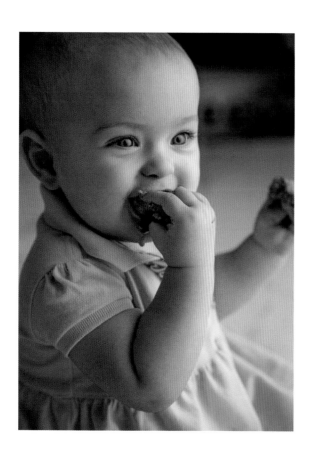

DONNA'S BASIC SANDWICH BREAD

YIELD: *1 medium sized loaf*

Babies and little kids can't handle the high levels of sodium that we are often accustomed to as adults. While keeping salt out of baby's diet is relatively simple when it comes to homemade purees, finding a great low-sodium sandwich bread can be challenging. Most breads sold at the grocery store are packed with sodium, not to mention plenty of other preservatives and additives that little ones don't really need in their developing bodies.

Making your own bread is a great solution, and the following recipe is simple enough to be prepared without special expertise or even a whole lot of effort. You can even freeze your fresh-baked loaves to make the most out of each bread-making session.

This recipe was shared with me by Donna Currie, a fellow food blogger (cookistry.com), author, and bread baking expert. When I asked Donna for a bread that would be easy to make and that would still come out well with a lower than usual amount of salt, she knew just what I needed. This bread is very easy to make, and should come together nicely for even the most inexperienced bakers.

INGREDIENTS

- 1 cup (240 ml) lukewarm water
- 1 tablespoon (15 g) white sugar
- 2¼ teaspoons (11.25 ml) / 1 package instant yeast
- 2½ cups (11¼ oz) all-purpose flour
- 1 teaspoon (5 g) salt
- 2 tablespoons (30 ml) olive oil
- Cornmeal for dusting

DIRECTIONS

1. Add the sugar and yeast to the water in your measuring cup and stir to combine.

2. Put the flour and salt into a medium bowl, and stir to distribute salt.

3. Add the water/yeast mixture to the bowl with the flour, and stir to combine all the ingredients.

4. Sprinkle some flour on your countertop and dump the dough mixture onto the counter. Knead for a minute or two, adding flour as necessary to keep it from sticking. You don't need to knead until the dough is stretchy and elastic—just knead until it's a nice cohesive mixture and not a lumpy, sticky, blobby mess. Form it into a ball.

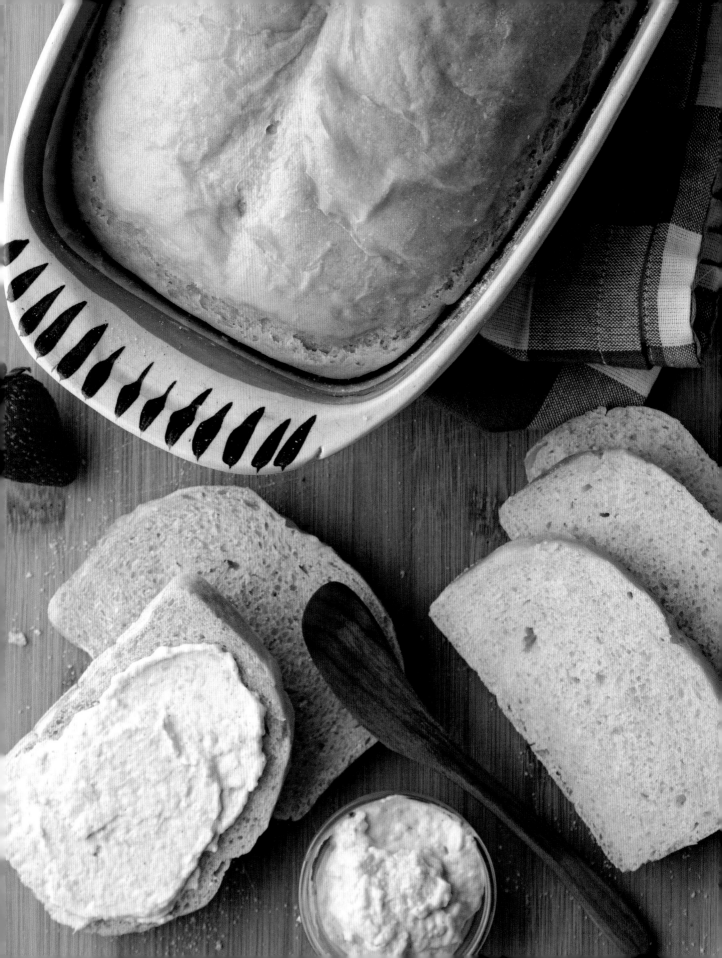

5. Drizzle the olive oil into a zip-top bag and plop the dough into the bag. Make sure the dough is completely coated with olive oil, zip the top, and stash it in the refrigerator overnight.

6. The next day, take the bag out of the fridge and massage the dough a bit while still in the bag to mash out all the bubbles. You may need to open the bag to let the air out, but reseal it after.

7. Leave the bag on the countertop until the dough has come to room temperature, about 1 hour. It will rise and expand a bit during that time.

8. Preheat the oven to 350°F (177°C). Sprinkle some cornmeal on the bottom of a loaf pan.

9. Sprinkle some flour on your countertop and dump the dough onto the counter. You don't need to squeeze every bit of olive oil out of the bag, but don't try to hold it back, either.

10. Knead and fold the dough a bit to incorporate the olive oil, then form the dough into a log that will fit into your loaf pan.

11. Put the loaf into the pan, cover the pan with plastic wrap, and let it rise until it has at least doubled in size. I used an 8½ x 4½-inch (22 x 11cm) pan and let it rise until it was slightly higher than the pan.

12. Remove the plastic wrap and slash the top.

13. Bake at 350°F (177°C) for 35 to 40 minutes, until the bread is golden brown and the loaf sounds hollow when tapped.

14. Let it rest in the pan for about 5 minutes, then place it on a rack to cool completely before slicing.

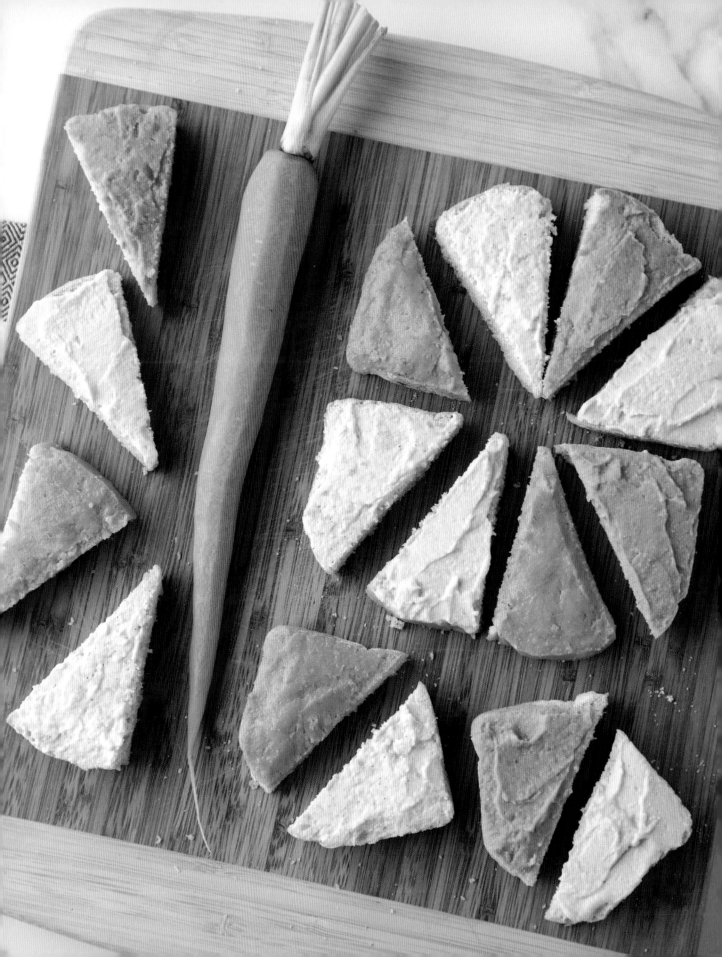

SAVORY SAMMIE SPREADS

Cute little sandwiches can be a wonderful vessel for a variety of healthy foods. Plus, they are great fun to grasp and smash, allowing babies to work on fine motor skills while enjoying their food. Try slicing sammies up into tiny squares, long rectangles, or classic triangles to give your little one plenty of new shapes to try out.

Spread a couple of tablespoons of one of the following spreads on Donna's basic sandwich bread (page 137) or slices of store-bought bread, tortillas, or pitas. When shopping for bread, look for varieties labeled as low sodium, or visit your local baker to see if they have any freshly baked low-sodium or gluten-free breads available.

The following recipes are easy to customize by replacing main ingredients with similar fruits, veggies, or beans. For example, you might try making this hummus recipe with black beans instead of chickpeas. Apple butter can be swapped for any type of low-sugar jam or jelly you like to customize the yogurt spread.

Your little one might love green pea guacamole with a little pureed spinach mixed in, and the cheese spread can easily be made with sweet potatoes or even cauliflower in place of carrots. Like baby purees, savory sammie spreads are made to be tailored to your own child's needs and preferences.

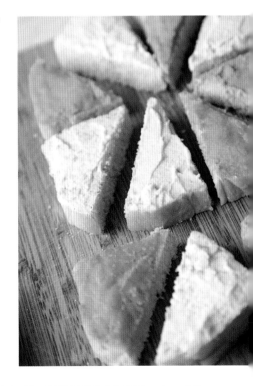

hummus

YIELD: *1½ cups (355 ml)*

DIRECTIONS

1. Place dried chickpeas in a small saucepan and cover with water. Pick out and discard any beans that float to the top. Bring water to a boil, then reduce to a simmer and cook, covered, for about 2 hours, or until the beans are soft enough to mash with a fork.

2. Drain chickpeas, reserving about ½ cup of the cooking liquid, then rinse. Allow chickpeas and reserved liquid to cool to the touch (about 15 minutes).

3. Combine chickpeas with lemon juice, olive oil, spices (if using), and 2 tablespoons of the reserved cooking liquid in food processor and pulse until well chopped. Add 2 more tablespoons cooking liquid and puree until smooth, adding more liquid as needed.

4. Store in an airtight resealable container for up to 2 weeks in the refrigerator or 3 months in the freezer.

INGREDIENTS

- 4 ounces (120 g) dried chickpeas
- 2 cups (480 ml) water
- 2 tablespoons (30 ml) lemon juice
- 2 tablespoons (30 ml) virgin olive oil
- ½ teaspoon (2.5 ml) garlic powder (optional)
- ¼ teaspoon (1.25 ml) onion powder (optional)

yogurt spread

YIELD: *½ cup (120 ml)*

DIRECTIONS

1. Mix yogurt and apple butter together in small mixing bowl.

2. Set a small colander lined with several layers of cheesecloth in a small mixing bowl. Pour yogurt into the colander and cover with tight lid or plastic or beeswax wrap.

3. Refrigerate for 24 hours, until the mixture becomes thick and creamy, like dip or cream cheese.

4. Transfer to a small resealable container and store in fridge for up to 1 week.

INGREDIENTS

- 4 ounces (120 ml) plain whole milk yogurt
- 2 tablespoons (30 ml) slow-cooked apple butter (page 131) or jam/jelly of choice

green pea guacamole

YIELD: *About ¾ cup (180 ml)*

DIRECTIONS

1. Combine avocado and green peas in a blender or food processor and puree until smooth, adding a splash of water if needed.

2. Add lime juice to taste and puree again to blend ingredients.

3. Store in airtight container with a small piece of waxed paper placed directly on the surface of the spread to help prevent browning. Can be refrigerated for up to 3 days or frozen for up to 3 months.

INGREDIENTS

» ½ cup (120 ml) ripe avocado (about ½ avocado)

» ¼ cup (60 ml) green peas

» Up to 1 tablespoon (15 ml) lime juice

carrot cheddar spread

YIELD: *1¼ cup (300 ml)*

DIRECTIONS

1. Place sliced carrots in small saucepan and cover with about 2 inches (50mm) water. Bring to a boil, then reduce to simmer and cook 10 to 15 minutes, or until carrots are soft enough to be mashed with a fork.

2. Drain carrots and rinse with cold water until they become cool to the touch.

3. Combine carrots, cheeses, butter, and spices (if using) in food processor or blender and puree until smooth.

4. Store in airtight container and refrigerate for up to 1 week or freeze for up to 3 months.

INGREDIENTS

» ½ cup (120 ml) carrots, sliced

» 4 ounces (120 g) mild cheddar cheese, shredded

» 4 ounces (120 g) mozzarella cheese, shredded

» 2 tablespoons (30 ml) unsalted butter, melted

» ½ teaspoon (2.5 ml) paprika (optional)

» ¼ teaspoon (1.25 ml) garlic powder (optional)

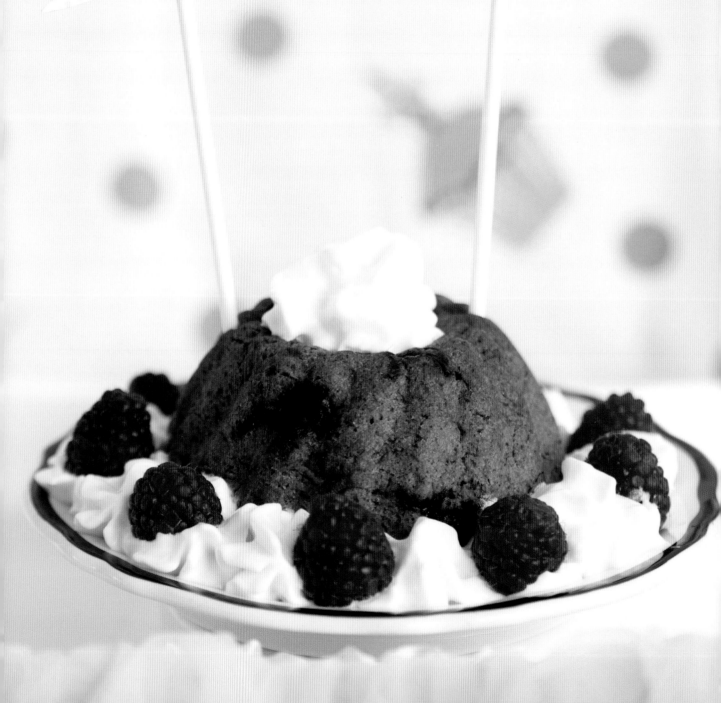

HEALTHY SMASH CAKE

YIELD: *2 small cakes*

One tradition that I dreaded upon my son's own first birthday was his first bite of cake. It's not that I'm opposed to a mess, or even my child getting his first real sugar rush. I might be kinda crunchy, but I'm really not *too* uptight. It was just kind of a bummer to have spent the last twelve months (well, more like twenty-two if you count pregnancy) fiercely defending this new life from things like synthetic chemicals, potential toxins, and sketchy foods only to plop him into a pile of hydrogenated oil, high fructose corn syrup, and food dye on his first birthday. As his party approached, I had my heart set on baking him a special healthy cake. But then life went upside-down (like it does) and I ran out of time to make it for him. We ended up getting a giant sheet cake from the local wholesale store—slathered in rainbow-colored frosting and sporting an ingredient list that I would have needed a magnifying glass to decipher.

Did we all survive? Yes. Did we sleep that night? No.

If I had that day to do over again, I would have baked him this cake. It's made with fruits and veggies and all-natural goodies! Mountainous peaks of freshly whipped cream give baby plenty of ammunition for creating that adorable mess we have all come to expect in first birthday photographs.

INGREDIENTS

- 1¼ cups (300 ml) all-purpose flour*
- ½ cup (120 ml) whole wheat flour*
- 1½ teaspoons (7.5 ml) baking soda
- ¼ cup (60 ml) carrot or sweet potato puree (recipe page 123)
- ¼ cup (60 ml) milk or plant-based milk
- ⅓ cup (80 ml) applesauce
- ½ cup (120 ml) sugar
- ⅓ cup (80 ml) cooking oil
- 1 banana, mashed
- 1 teaspoon (5 ml) lemon juice
- 1 teaspoon (5 ml) vanilla extract
- 1 cup (240 ml) blueberries

For Topping

- ½ cup (120 ml) heavy whipping cream
- 1 tablespoon (15 ml) powdered sugar
- ½ cup (120 ml) fresh blueberries
- ½ cup (120 ml) fresh raspberries

*For a gluten-free cake, substitute these flours with 1 ¾ cups (420 ml) all-purpose gluten-free flour (recipe page 30).

HEALTHY SMASH CAKE *(continued)*

DIRECTIONS

1. Preheat oven to 325°F (163°C). Grease two miniature Bundt pans or 4" (10cm) cake pans with butter or cooking oil.

2. In a large mixing bowl, whisk together the flours and baking soda.

3. In a second bowl, combine the carrot or sweet potato puree, milk, applesauce, sugar, cooking oil, mashed banana, lemon juice, and vanilla extract. Whisk until fairly smooth.

4. Add the liquid ingredients to the dry, and then mix until well combined. Gently fold in blueberries, then pour into cake pans.

5. Bake for 40 to 45 minutes,* or until firm and golden brown. To test for doneness, stick a dry toothpick in the center of the cake. When the toothpick comes out clean, the cake is done.

6. Allow the cakes to cool in their pans for 30 minutes before turning them out onto cooling racks.

7. To make whipped cream, combine heavy whipping cream and powdered sugar and whisk with electric mixer for several minutes at the highest speed, or until the cream forms soft peaks that easily hold their shape. Store whipped cream in the refrigerator until cake is served.

8. When cakes have cooled completely, top with whipped cream and fresh berries just before serving.

*If using gluten-free flour, bake for an extra 10 to 15 minutes.

handmade mama tip

CUSTOMIZING THE SMASH CAKE

If you have your heart set on colored frosting, try adding a few teaspoons of pureed strawberries, blueberries, or a dash of turmeric powder to the cream as it is being whipped. This will impart a subtle touch of color to make your cake a little more festive. You can also find natural food dye recommendations in the appendix on page 194.

This cake can easily be made to accommodate a range of dietary concerns, allergies, or intolerances. Just swap the flours for gluten-free types, and use your favorite plant-based milk for cow's milk. Even the pureed carrot can be swapped out for another sweet pureed fruit or veggie, like sweet potato or extra applesauce. Not a fan of blueberries? Try using chopped strawberries, raisins, or even chocolate chips instead. Just keep in mind that these changes might alter the baking time slightly.

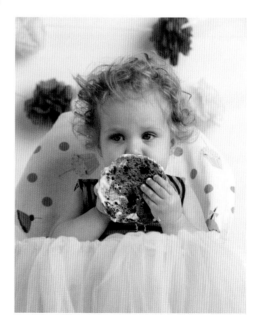

BURP CLOTHS

YIELD: *4 burp cloths*

Babies are messy creatures. No matter how fastidious they may one day grow to be, babies are sure to spend their early days dribbling, drooling, and burping with the best of them. It helps to have plenty of spittle control gear on hand, and the best item in your baby arsenal is the mighty burp cloth.

These simple cloths can be made in large batches, and depending on the fabric you choose, they can be as cutesy or minimalist as you like. They are also great for gifting, since they can easily be personalized to suit a mama's style or match a nursery theme.

This project makes four burp cloths at a time. Trust me when I tell you that you can't have too many. When my son was an infant, I kept a fresh pile of burp cloths by the rocker, another on the arm of our couch, and an extra stash next to my bed. Anywhere baby and I had a habit of sitting down, there was a burp cloth at the ready.

MATERIALS + TOOLS

- 1 yard (91cm) flannel
- 1 yard (91cm) cotton batting
- Matching thread
- Cereal bowl or other round object
- Scissors or a rotary cutter with mat
- Pins
- Ruler or measuring tape
- Sewing machine

DIRECTIONS

1. Measure and cut six 10 x 18-inch (25.5 x 46cm) rectangles of fabric and three 10 x 20-inch (25.5 x 51cm) of batting.

2. Place two fabric rectangles on a flat surface with right sides together and one layer of batting on top. Use a cereal bowl or other round object to trace round quarter-circles on each corner. Cut round edges off rectangles, using traced shape (see figure 1, page 149).

3. Pin and stitch around edges, leaving one 2-inch (5cm) opening to turn out fabric (see figure 2, page 149).

4. Turn out fabric and hand-stitch the opening closed (instructions on pages 19–20).

5. Sew a stitch about ¼-inch (6mm) around the inner edge of the burp cloths to give them a sturdy, finished edge (see figure 3, page 149).

6. Repeat steps 1 to 5 three times to make three more burp cloths.

TO USE

Drape over your shoulder to catch spit-up, or keep one handy to wipe up spills.

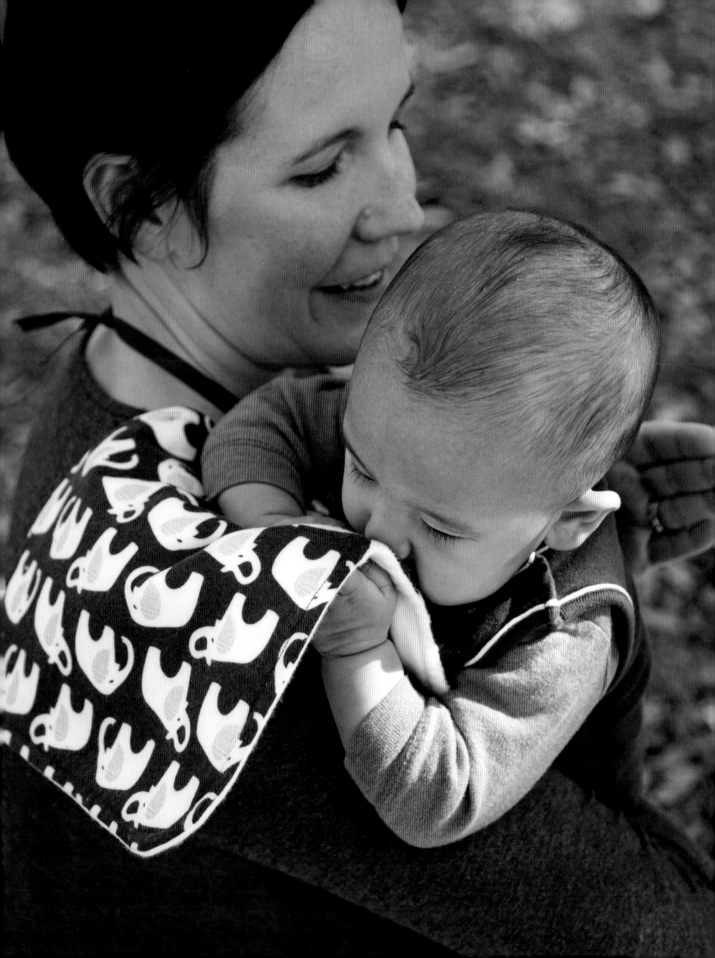

BURP CLOTHS *(continued)*

Figure 1

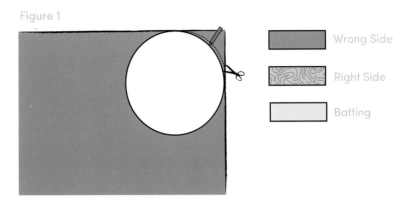

▒▒	Wrong Side
░░	Right Side
□	Batting

Figure 2

Figure 3

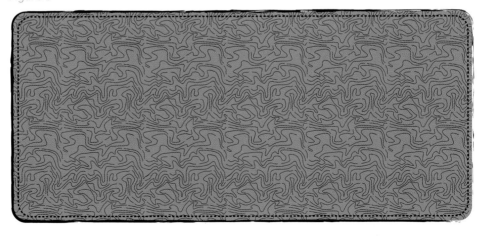

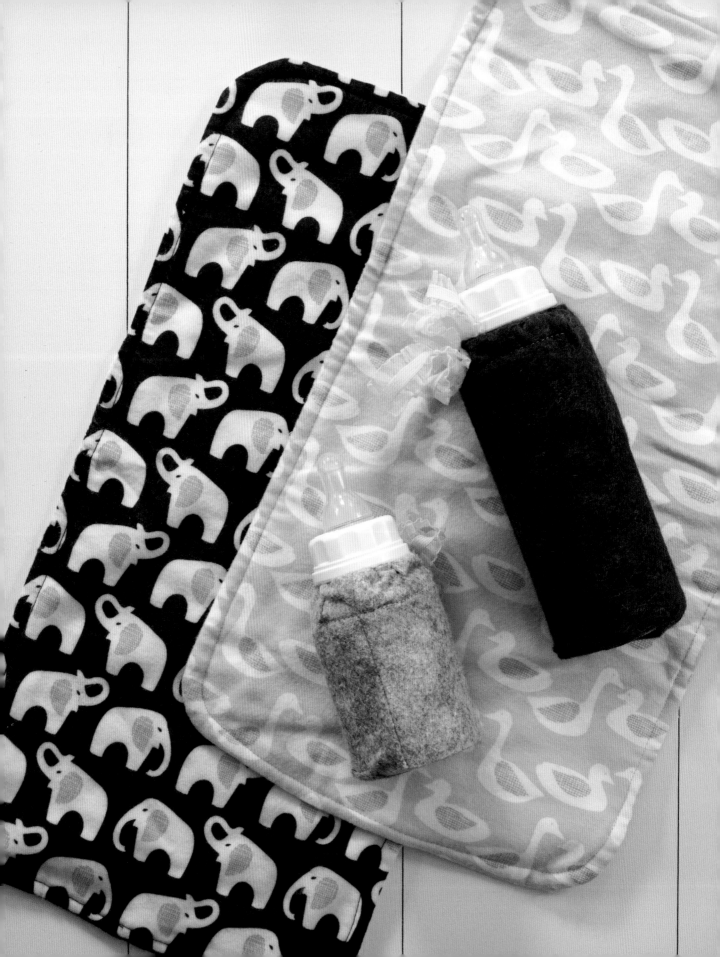

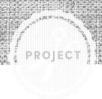
BOTTLE COZIES

YIELD: *4 bottle cozies*

MATERIALS + TOOLS

- ½ yard (46cm) wool felt
- 4 12-in. (30.5cm) pieces of fold-over elastic
- Matching thread
- Scissors or a rotary cutter with mat
- Pins
- Ruler or measuring tape
- Sewing machine
- Safety pin

Milk goes cold when it should be warm and gets warm when you want to keep it cold. Sometimes I wonder if the originator of Murphy's Law had children. Papa (or perhaps) Mama Murphy may have found the idea of a baby bottle cozy quite handy—especially if they had a particularly finicky baby. Some little ones demand their milk at a very specific temperature; these woolen cozies should keep the bottle right on target as baby chugs it down.

Because baby bottles come in lots of different shapes and sizes, you will need to measure your own bottles to provide a custom fit.

DIRECTIONS

Measure and Cut Pattern Pieces

1. Measure the height (from bottom to neck) of the bottle you are using. Add 1½ inches (38mm) to this measurement and write down the total as Measurement 1.

2. Measure around the widest point of the bottle. Add ¾ inch (19cm) to this measurement and write down the total as Measurement 2.

3. Measure across the bottom of the bottle to get its width. Add ¼ inch (6mm) to this measurement and write down the total as Measurement 3.

4. To make the Piece As, cut four pieces of felt using Measurements 1 and 2 as the height and width (Measurement 1 x Measurement 2).

5. To make the Piece Bs, cut four pieces of felt using Measurement 3 as the length and using 1 inch (2.5cm) as the width.

Assemble Bottle Cozies

6. Fold each Piece A in half by its width and pin side edges. Sew up the side of the piece, leaving the top and bottom open (see figure 1, page 152).

7. Fold the top edge of the piece down by 1 inch (2.5cm) to form a hem. Sew around the inner edge of the hem to form a tube around the top of the piece (see figure 2, page 152).

8. Turn the piece right-side out.

9. Pin one short side of a Piece B to the bottom of each cozy. Sew the short side onto the bottom using a ⅛-inch (3mm) seam allowance (see figure 3, page 152).

10. Pin and sew the other short side of Piece B onto the opposite side of the cozy's bottom edge.

Finish Cozy

11. Snip four evenly spaced notches into the top hem, stopping just before the hem seam (see figure 4, below).

12. Attach a safety pin to one end of the fold-over elastic and thread it through the top hem of the cozy.

13. Slip the cozy over a bottle and pull the elastic snugly. Tie a small knot in the elastic. The elastic should be tight enough to keep the cozy in place but loose enough to stretch easily for removal.

14. Snip excess elastic from top.

TO USE

Slip over a bottle after getting it to the proper temperature for baby.

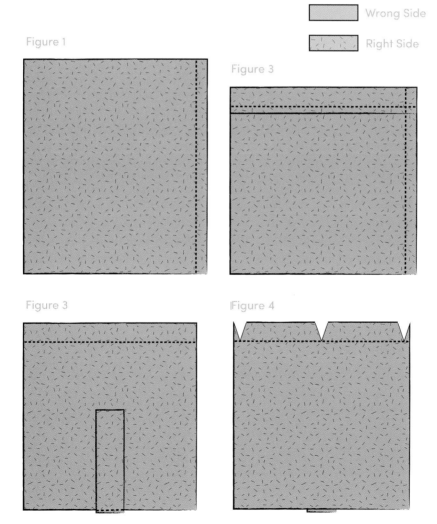

Wrong Side

Right Side

Figure 1

Figure 3

Figure 3

Figure 4

TERRYCLOTH TEETHERS

YIELD: *2 terrycloth teethers*

Little ones aren't usually very happy when they are cutting new teeth. Sore gums can give even the sweetest little pumpkin a cranky attitude, and those new chompers can take a toll on mom and dad's patience too.

Having something handy to gnaw on can help take the edge off pain and discomfort during teething. Like everything else, babies tend to have preferences when it comes to teethers. Some kids love chomping on wooden rings, while others prefer icy plastic teethers or silicone shapes. You can even find teethers made from leather.

My son really loved teethers made from terrycloth. These simple cloth teethers can be soaked in water and chilled or enjoyed temporarily dry. (Baby will drool some moisture into them shortly.) I made two different vegetable shapes for this project. Feel free to swap out the colors to make your own favorite veggies like carrots, beets, rutabagas, and daikon radish.

MATERIALS + TOOLS

- ¼ yard (23cm) terrycloth
- Tracing paper and pencil
- Matching thread
- Pins
- Ruler or measuring tape
- Sewing machine

DIRECTIONS

Cut Pattern Pieces

1. Cut or trace pattern pieces (Terrycloth Teether A, Terrycloth Teether B, Terrycloth Teether C) from pattern library (page 190).

2. Fold terrycloth in half. Pin pattern pieces to fabric and cut.

Make Stem

3. Match both pairs of Terrycloth Teether C pieces, right sides together, and pin edges.

4. Sew around edges of each pair using a ⅛-inch (3mm) seam allowance, leaving the bottom of the stem open for turning out (see figure 1, page 155).

5. Turn out both Terrycloth Teether C pieces (instructions on page 20).

Make Teether A and B

6. Match two Terrycloth Teether A pieces, right sides together, and pin edges. Place one finished Terrycloth Teether C piece between the two A pieces at the top of the vegetable. The raw edge should be sticking out about 1 inch (2.5cm) with the finished side sandwiched between the two pieces (see figure 2, page 155).

7. Sew around edges using a ⅛-inch (3mm) seam allowance, leaving a 2-inch (5cm) opening for turning out (see figure 2, page 155).

8. Repeat with pieces of Terrycloth Teether B.

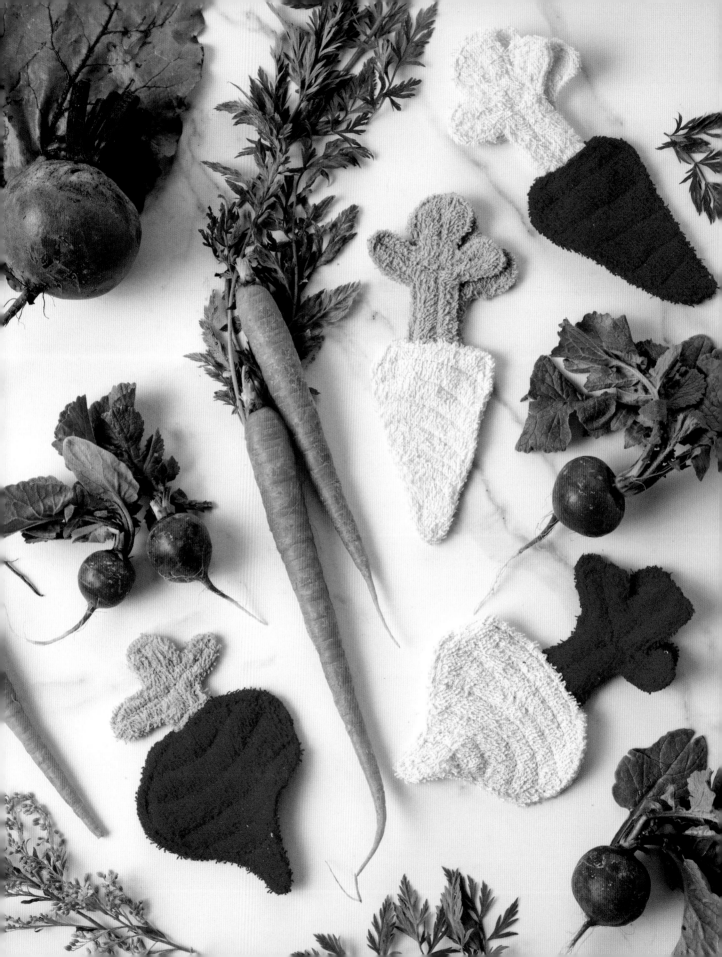

TERRYCLOTH TEETHERS *(continued)*

Finish Teethers

9. Turn out both teethers and hand-stitch openings closed (instructions on pages 19–20).

10. Using coordinating thread, stitch around the edges of the finished teethers to give them detail and structure. Also stitch stripes into the body and leaves of each teether (see figure 3, below).

TO USE

Share with baby dry or soaked with chilled water. Launder as needed and remove any dangling threads if necessary.

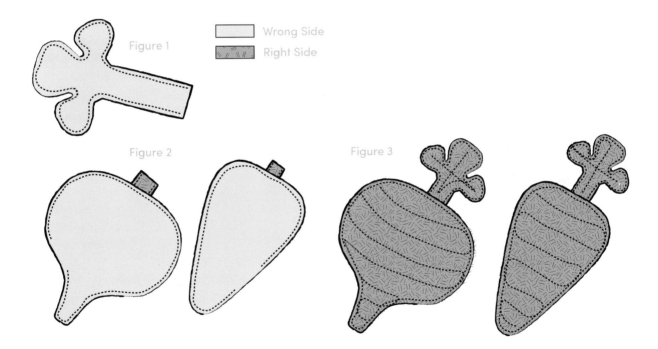

Figure 1

Wrong Side
Right Side

Figure 2

Figure 3

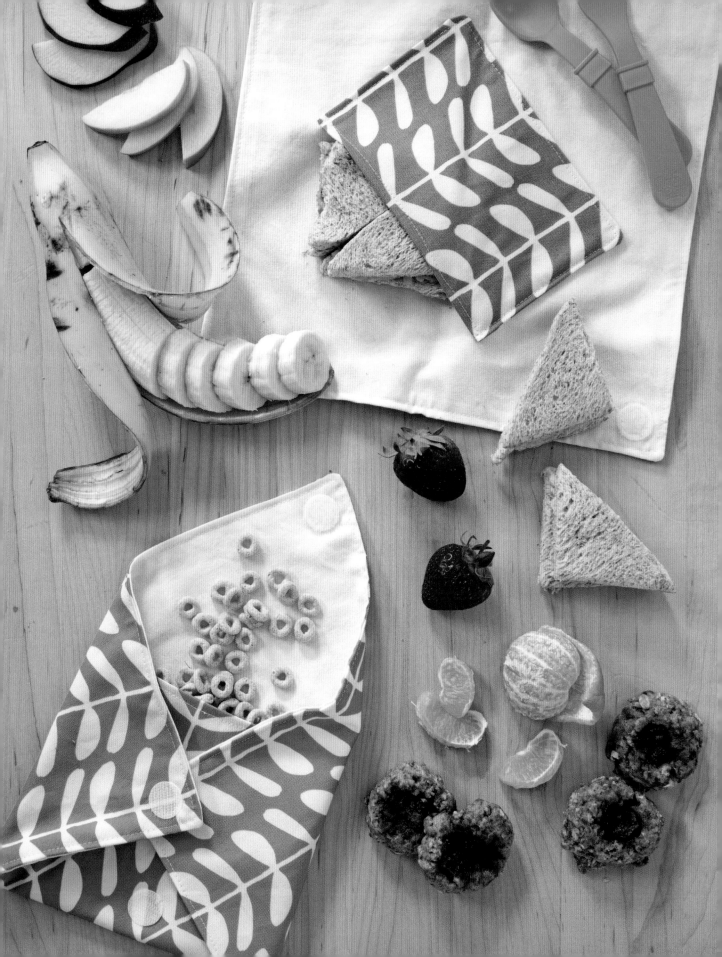

SARAH'S SNACK ENVELOPE

YIELD: *1 snack envelope*

My sister, Sarah, is the real sewing dynamo in our family (she can make anything from costumes to baby clothes like a pro). When I decided to include sewing projects in this book, I really hoped that Sarah would share a pattern. I knew whatever she came up with would be special and she did not disappoint! This clever snack holder doubles as a placemat, granting both you and baby the freedom to snack whenever and wherever you happen to be. As someone whose child has inherited the "hangry" gene, I find that feature extremely attractive! The following is from Sarah:

This cute envelope-style pouch is a quick sew and a handy accessory in any mama's bag! With an inner pocket and adjustable hook-and-loop closures, you can store treats galore inside. Open just the top flap to store snacks, or unfold the entire piece to reveal a handy mat (a nice bonus when you're out and about). My favorite part of this pouch is that it's sized generously enough to fit a sandwich—extending its usefulness past the land of puffs and cookies.

If you're looking for water resistance, you can certainly substitute fabric, but please be sure that it is food safe. Oil cloth, for example, is waterproof and comes in very appealing prints, but is *not* food safe. Waxed canvas (no lining would be necessary) or Eco-PUL (used as a lining with a cotton woven outer) are both food-safe, water-resistant options.

MATERIALS + TOOLS

- ½ yard (46cm) cotton canvas, main color
- ½ yard (46cm) cotton canvas, contrasting color
- 5 sets ¾-in. (20mm) sew-on round hook-and-loop closures (3 sets plus 2 additional hook closures)
- Matching thread
- Scissors or a rotary cutter with mat
- Pins
- Ruler or measuring tape
- Sewing machine

DIRECTIONS

Note: The seam allowance for this project is ⅜-inch (9.5mm) unless otherwise noted.

Measure and Cut Pieces

1. Measure and cut one 11 x 11-inch (28 x 28cm) piece and one 8½ x 6½-inch (22 x 15cm) piece in the main color.

2. Measure and cut one 11 x 11-inch (28 x 28cm) piece from the contrasting color fabric.

SARAH'S SNACK ENVELOPE *(continued)*

Create the Envelope

3. Place the 11-inch (28cm) square pieces together, right sides facing, and pin at the edges, leaving a 2-inch (5cm) opening for turning (see figure 1, page 159).

4. Stitch together, making sure not to stitch over the opening you made.

5. Clip the corners close to the stitching and turn the piece right side out (instructions on page 20).

6. Press flat; fold the seam allowance of the opening in and press.

7. Topstitch the entire piece with a ¼-inch (6mm) seam allowance, stitching the opening closed as you do this (see figure 2, page 159).

Make Inner Pocket

8. Cut an 8½ x 6½-inch (22 x 15cm) piece from main fabric for the inner pocket.

9. Fold piece in half with right sides facing and pin at edges, leaving a 2-inch (5cm) opening for turning (see figure 3, page 159).

10. Stitch the pocket together at the sides, making sure not to stitch over the opening.

11. Clip the corners and turn the piece right side out.

12. Press flat; fold the seam allowance of the opening in and press.

13. Topstitch the top edge with a ¼-inch (6mm) seam allowance (see figure 4, page 159).

Attach Pocket

14. Position the envelope like a diamond. Fold the piece in half widthwise and mark the center either with a disappearing ink pen or by finger pressing a crease in the fabric. Repeat by folding the piece in half widthwise.

15. Mark the center of the inner pocket using the same method.

16. Position the pocket in the center of the envelope by lining up your center marks. Pin in place.

17. Stitch a ¼-inch (6mm) seam around the three outer edges of the pocket, leaving the top edge open (see figure 5, page 159).

Attach Hook-and-Loop Tape

18. Stitch loop (fuzzy) pieces to the top, left, and right corners of the interior envelope as shown in the diagram (see figure 6, page 159). Be sure to back stitch on all hook-and-loop pieces as they will be getting a lot of wear and tear!

19. Stitch hook (scratchy) pieces to the left, right, and bottom corners of the exterior envelope as shown in the diagram (see figure 7, page 159).

TO USE

Fold the corners in until they overlap. The three hook pieces on the bottom corner allow you to adjust the fit to the size of the contents. Fold and fill (and wash) often!

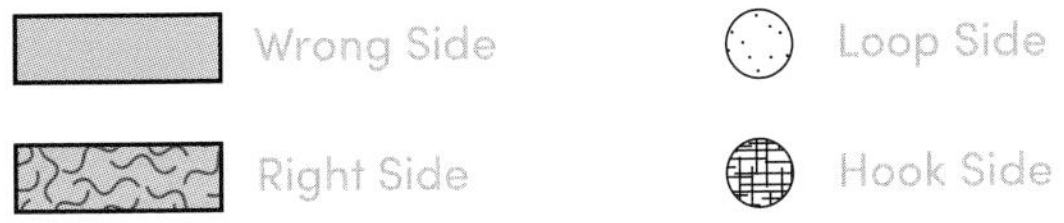

	Wrong Side		Loop Side
	Right Side		Hook Side

Figure 1

Figure 2

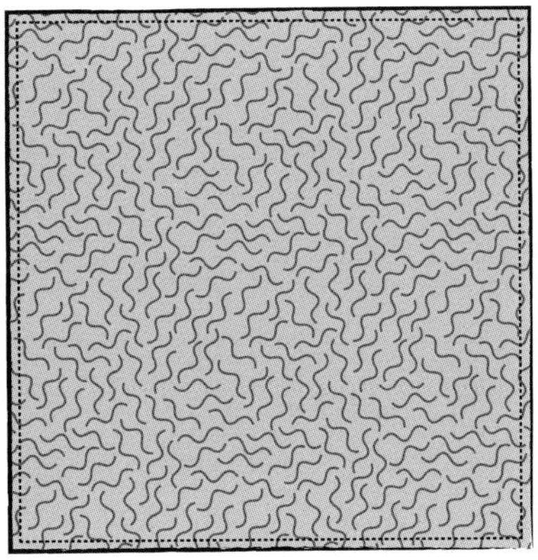

Figure 3

Figure 4

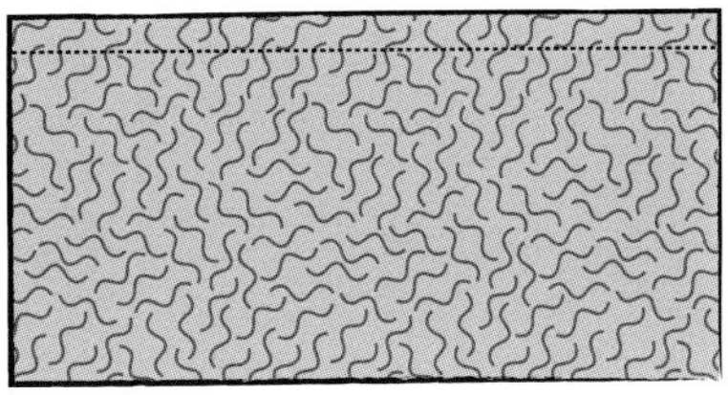

Figure 5

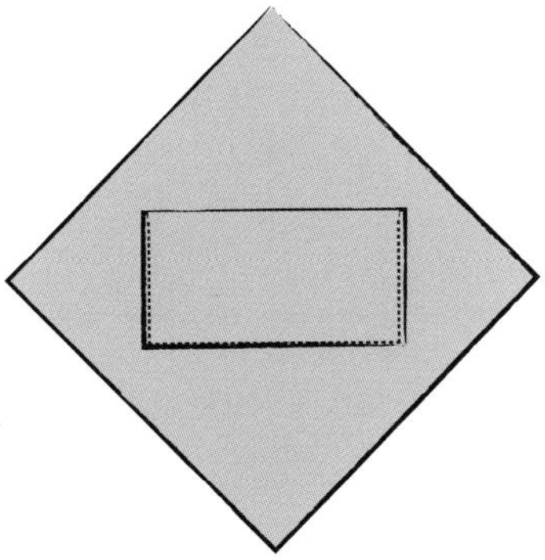

Figure 6

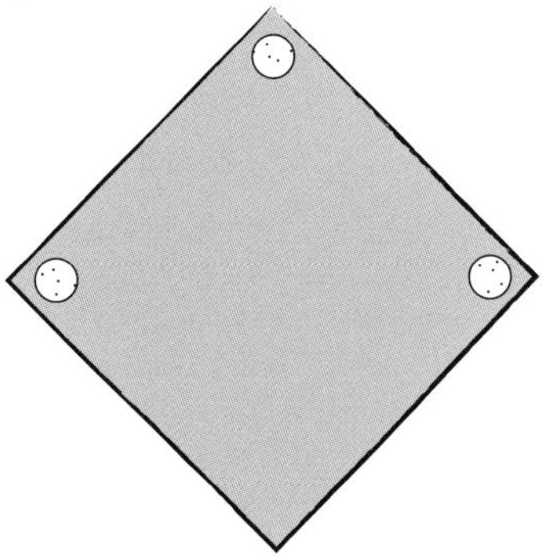

Figure 7

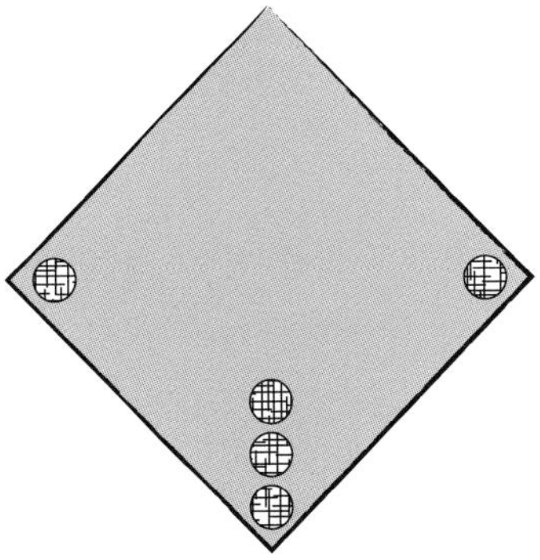

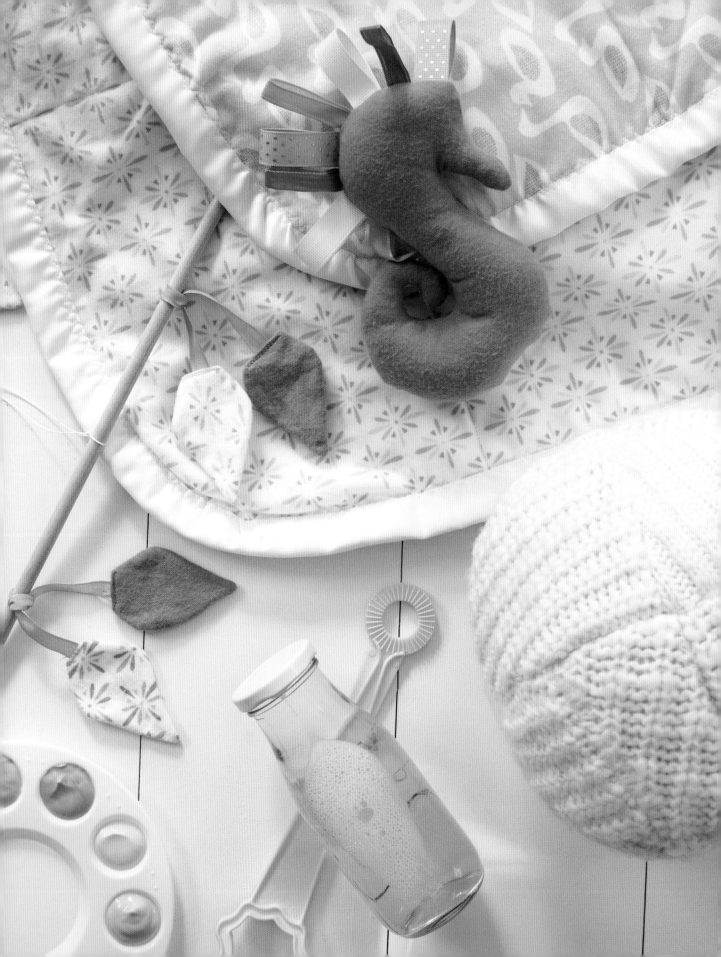

↡

chapter 5

PLAYTIME

Fred Rogers said, "Play is often talked about as if it were a relief from serious learning. But for children, play is serious learning. Play is really the work of childhood." Even from babyhood, little ones are building important connections and flexing their intellectual muscles through play. Every new sensation, intriguing sound, and object of beauty is a learning opportunity.

Besides, there isn't much better in the whole wide world than watching your child discover and delight in something new. Watching their little eyes light up, seeing their smiles, and hearing the sound of their laughter makes encouraging play a rewarding experience for both of you.

In this chapter, I share recipes and projects for making playtime both fun and enriching. From making a mess with sensory play to chasing bubbles, babies and toddlers are constantly working on developing their sensory systems, motor skills, and cognitive abilities while they appear to be simply having fun. The brain uses these experiences to lay foundations and make connections that your child will depend on for an entire lifetime. No pressure, right?

Luckily, babies and children are hardwired to crave the kind of input that hands-on play provides. All you have to do is create opportunities for your child to have fun. Let baby get his hands dirty. Encourage your little one to reach out and touch something new or make a closer inspection of a favorite toy. Allow satisfaction of curiosity through exploration and discovery. The brilliant baby brain will do the rest. ➡

what is sensory play?

Young children and babies often have strong reactions to different kinds of textures or sounds. Some babies love squishing food through their fingers, while others can't stand having their hands dirty. A funny-sounding rattle might make one baby laugh, but frighten the next. These reactions offer adults a window into our children's sensory experience, which is likely to be much different than our own.

The body's sensory systems help us to interpret everything from temperature and texture to our body's own position in space or sense of motion. These senses have strong ties with our motor skills, our speech, and even basic functions like sleeping and eating. In a way, our sensory system acts like a guide, helping us to navigate the world around us using a vast library within our brains.

Take a moment to imagine what it must be like to experience life without a complete sensory library. That thought may come in handy while trying to understand why a child melts down over their food being hot instead of cold, or discovering an itchy tag on their new favorite pair of pajamas. Not only are their minds still learning how to navigate this big new world, their bodies are too.

For this library to function at its best, it requires lots and lots of input. Every time your child hears, sees, tastes, touches, or smells something new, the brain is gobbling up that information and putting it to work in the sensory system. Giving babies and kids plenty of opportunities to experience new sensations is not only helpful to their development, but can also quite a bit of fun.

making mountains out of milestones

When I was pregnant with Charlie, I had a little app on my phone that would chime every week to tell me what size fruit he'd gotten to or which of his vital organs had developed that week. After he was born, it was hard to kick the habit of constantly checking to see if he measured up against the norm. I worried when he didn't smile right away, obsessed over whether he would roll over by a certain age, and fretted about the way he let one of his legs flop along while learning to crawl. Eventually I figured out that babies develop at their own pace and are unlikely to stick to a pre-determined timeline. For every milestone he hit early, he would hit another late. For every early climber we met, we'd befriend another child who simply refused to crawl. The truth is that babies are all different, and the older they get the further they tend to stray from a predictable milestone schedule. Of course, if you really feel like something isn't right, it's a good idea to trust your gut and ask an expert. A good pediatrician should always be there to give you a reality check, or if needed, the tools to address any delays that your child actually does encounter.

STAGES OF PLAY: HANDS-ON TOYS AND ACTIVITIES FOR EVERY AGE

AGE GROUP	TOYS	ACTIVITIES
0–3 months	Soft rattles and squeaky plushes; ribbon softies; baby play gym; black & white contrast card	Listening to voices; touching new objects; observing contrasting colors and shapes; reaching toward objects
3–6 months	Soft picture books; chewy squeak toys; activity balls; textured soft toys	Reading books; singing songs; swinging; peek-a-boo
6–9 months	Jumpers / exersaucers; baby piano / keyboard; nesting / stacking cups; simple musical instruments	Clapping and rhyming songs; banging and hammering; stacking and building blocks; rolling a ball
9–12 months	Light blocks; busy boards; toys with wheels; push toys; play tunnel; play silks	Crawling and cruising; singing and dancing; obstacle courses; chasing and hiding; building and arranging

the power of simple playthings

Every day we're surrounded by things that beep and chime, blink and light up, and blast us with noise and color. It can be a lot to take in as an adult. For little ones, whose sensory systems are still developing, the stimulus of the world around them can quickly feel overwhelming. By keeping playthings simple during baby's first year, you allow your child a slightly more gentle transition into this bright and noisy world. As baby grows older and the imagination blooms, you'll discover that something as simple as a wooden doll or a set of blocks can transform into anything desired. Not every toy in our home is battery-free (not by a long shot), but I love seeing my child focus on toys that encourage creativity and imagination through sheer simplicity.

get outside: tips on exploring the outdoors with little ones

As soon as you and your little one feel up to it, spending time outside can be a beautiful thing. Fresh air, sunshine, and a change of scenery can do a lot for boosting your mood, refreshing your energy, and preserving sanity after being cooped up with a newborn for any length of time. Oh yes, and it's good for baby too. Even very tiny babies can benefit from a walk with mama. Indirect sunlight can help baby soak up vitamin D, and babies often find the gentle motion of being securely carried or worn by mama or pushed in a stroller to be quite soothing. Like pretty much everything else to do with babies, clocking outside time may seem daunting at first. The following tips can help make getting out there a little bit easier.

INVEST IN GEAR THAT WORKS FOR YOU

Babies grow quickly, and whether you are pushing them or wearing them, comfort and safety are key. If you are using a stroller, make sure that your child is old enough to ride in it safely before going for a cruise. Look for a model that allows you to adjust the handles to account for your height, and pay close attention to how heavy or cumbersome the stroller is to stow and transport.

EMBRACE BABYWEARING

Baby carriers offer a range of comfort and versatility that strollers have a hard time matching. Once you find the carrier you like best and master the basics of getting baby in and out quickly, you can go pretty much anywhere without having to worry about whether your stroller tires can handle the terrain. There is a bit of a learning curve involved with some carriers—particularly the simpler styles like wraps and slings—but luckily, there are lots of generous babywearing mamas out there sharing their wisdom through Web sites and community groups. Check out the appendix on page 193 for a list of babywearing resources.

SCOPE OUT YOUR DESTINATION

If you are trying out a new hiking trail or park, finding out a few details before you arrive can be really helpful. How far is the location from your home? How long

---

ASK AN *expert*

Q: **What are your favorite games to play with infants?**

A: I don't know that you could call it a game, but I love talking to infants! Speaking with babies is vital to their language, social, and emotional development from the very beginning—even when it doesn't seem so because they can't respond.

—*Stacie Billis, food editor & cookbook author, eats.coolmompicks.com*

---

will it take to complete a loop on the trail, and what kind of terrain does it offer? Are there bathrooms available?

PLAN OUTINGS AROUND NAP TIMES

This is a tricky one, but if you can manage to time your outing just right, you can enjoy the great outdoors with a content or even sleeping baby. If baby is likely to be awake during your journey, an earlier outing will likely be the easiest. If you'd like to try to get your little one to sleep during the trip, try to start out right before their usual nap time.

CONNECT WITH YOUR COMMUNITY

You can combine your social time with outside time by finding community groups that focus on spending time outdoors. Look for playgroups or exercise groups using social media tools like Facebook Groups or Meetup.com, or suggest a

PERSONAL STORY

babies love books

I thought my Mom was a little nuts when she handed me and my two-month-old baby a book with the suggestion for me to read it to him. I wasn't entirely sure he could even see the pages yet. But she insisted that it was never too early to read to a child and even claimed that he would enjoy hearing the rhythm of my voice as I read the story aloud. Do you know what? She was right. He loved reading books! He loved reaching out his little baby hands toward the colorful pictures, and he cooed with joy as I softly spoke the words. He especially loved anything that rhymed. While our baby book reading sessions were a joy in and of themselves, the big payoff came later. Though my son has boundless energy and the attention span of any typical two-year-old (meaning, *very short*) he will still happily sit down with me and read book after book after book. It's a welcome respite from his usual breakneck pace, and I'm crossing my fingers that his love of reading will stay with him as he grows into an adult. For an unabashed bookworm like myself, I see that as the greatest reward of all.

group hike or outdoor picnic with parents you already know. Be sure to check out national organizations, like Hike It Baby, Fit4Mom, and Baby Boot Camp to find groups and events in your area.

PACK LIGHT

While you don't want to be encumbered by a heavy load, it's important to bring along what you need to accommodate baby's basic needs. I suggest putting together a mini diaper bag with just enough baby supplies to get through your hike. For me, that was one diaper, a handful of wipes, a simple change of clothes, and maybe a bottle or snack.

COVER UP

Pediatricians usually advise waiting until babies are at least six months old before using sunscreen or bug repellent (see page 90). Even then, I'm super-picky about what I use and how I use it. Before babies are ready for sunscreen and bug spray, their main defense is a physical barrier. Make sure baby has plenty of shade on the journey and is dressed with as much coverage as possible.

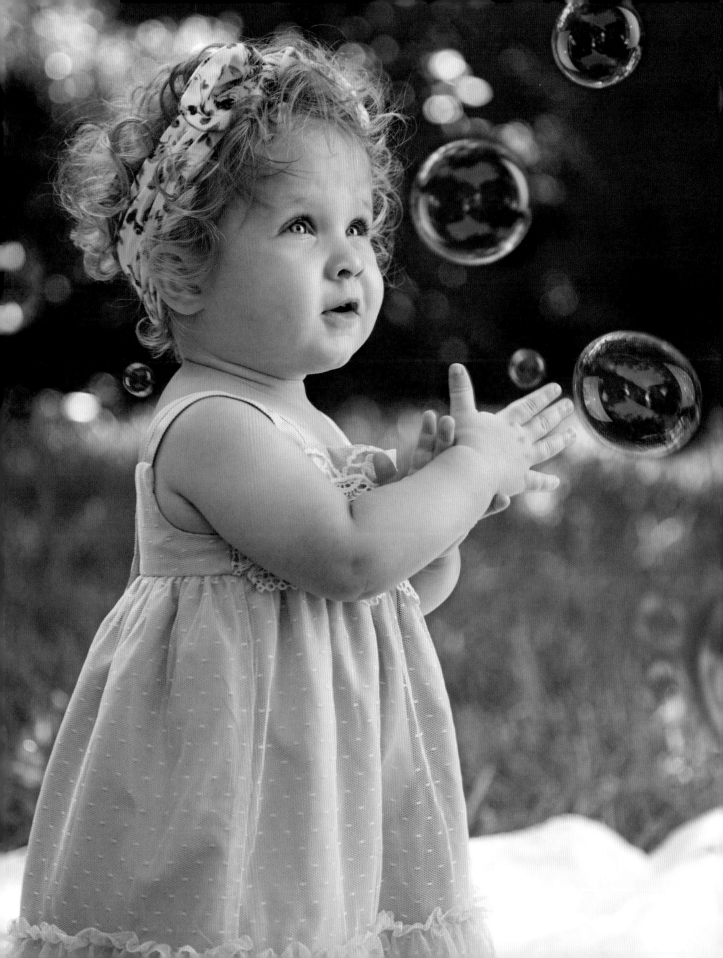

HOMEMADE BUBBLE SOLUTION

YIELD: 2 cups (480 ml)

Have you ever taken a close look at a soap bubble? It's a marvelous wonder of both nature and science—a perfect spherical orb contained only by the grace of its surface tension. Rainbows wink and shine along its slimy outer shell as it glides through the air on the whim of the breeze.

Of course, your wee one will probably not voice their adoration for bubbles with quite so many words, but believe me, baby *will* be impressed! Chasing bubbles is one of the quintessential and iconic thrills of childhood. It's a shame that the ingredient lists of most pre-packaged bubbles seem dubious at best.

If your child turns out to be anything like mine, he is likely to swallow as many bubbles as he catches—and exorbitantly more than he manages to blow! I started to wonder how easy it would be to make my own bubble solution and quickly found an Internet teeming with recipes to choose from. After some trial and error, I settled on the following recipe as my personal favorite. It is easy to make, requires no cooking, settling, or curing, and creates a modest, but altogether lovable bubble.

INGREDIENTS

- 1½ cups (360 ml) distilled water
- ½ cup (120 ml) unscented liquid dish soap
- ¾ teaspoon (3.75 ml) glycerin

Note: For children older than two, you can replace the glycerin with 3 tablespoons (45 ml) light corn syrup or honey.

DIRECTIONS

1. Combine ingredients in a small mixing bowl and stir together, slowly, until the liquids dissolve evenly.

TO USE

Dip bubble wand into solution, then blow gently to create bubbles. Solution should be refrigerated when not in use and stored for up to 3 weeks.

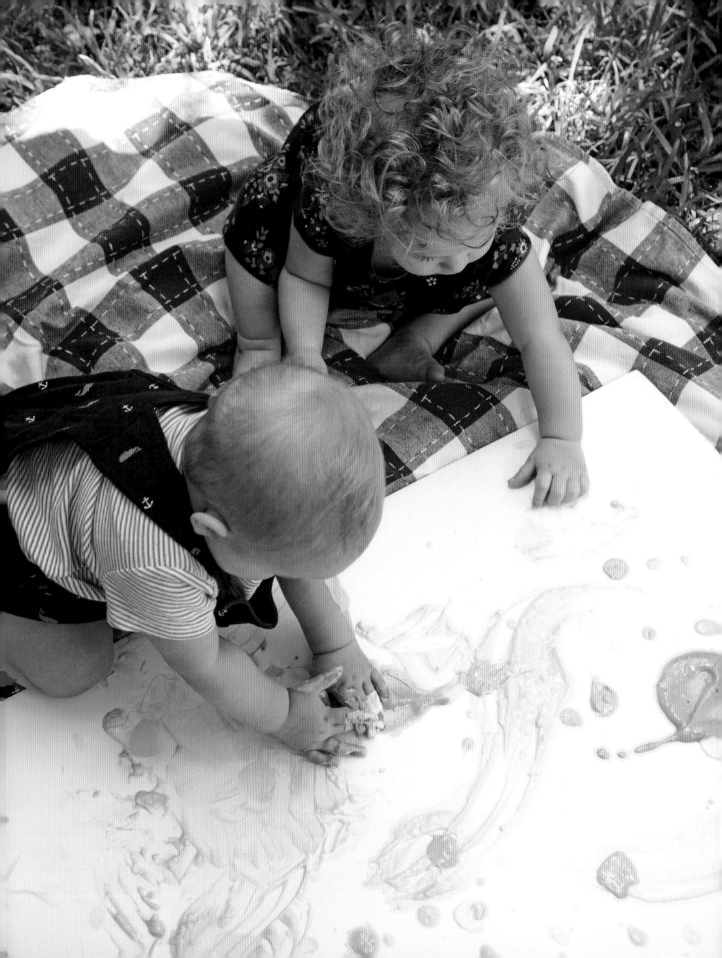

YOGURT FINGER PAINTS

YIELD: *1 cup (240 ml)*

If you have one of those kids who just can't resist putting anything and everything in their mouths, than you will love this totally edible alternative finger paint. Your little one's masterpiece may not stand the test of time, but she will have loads of fun blending, smearing, and perhaps also tasting this colorful goop. You'll find some recommended sources for plant-based food dyes in the resource section on page 194.

DIRECTIONS

1. Divide yogurt into three small bowls of ⅓ cup (80 ml) each.
2. Add a few drops of natural dye to each bowl, mixing well to blend in the color.
3. Refrigerate for up to 7 days.

TO USE

Cover baby's clothes in a smock or better yet, allow painting in the nude. Give baby a large piece of paper and start things off by dropping a few globs of colored "paint" onto the paper. Encourage baby to mash, smear, and smack the paint all over the page.

INGREDIENTS

- 1 cup (240 ml) plain whole milk yogurt, divided
- Natural food dye, as needed

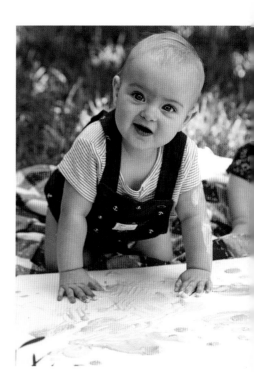

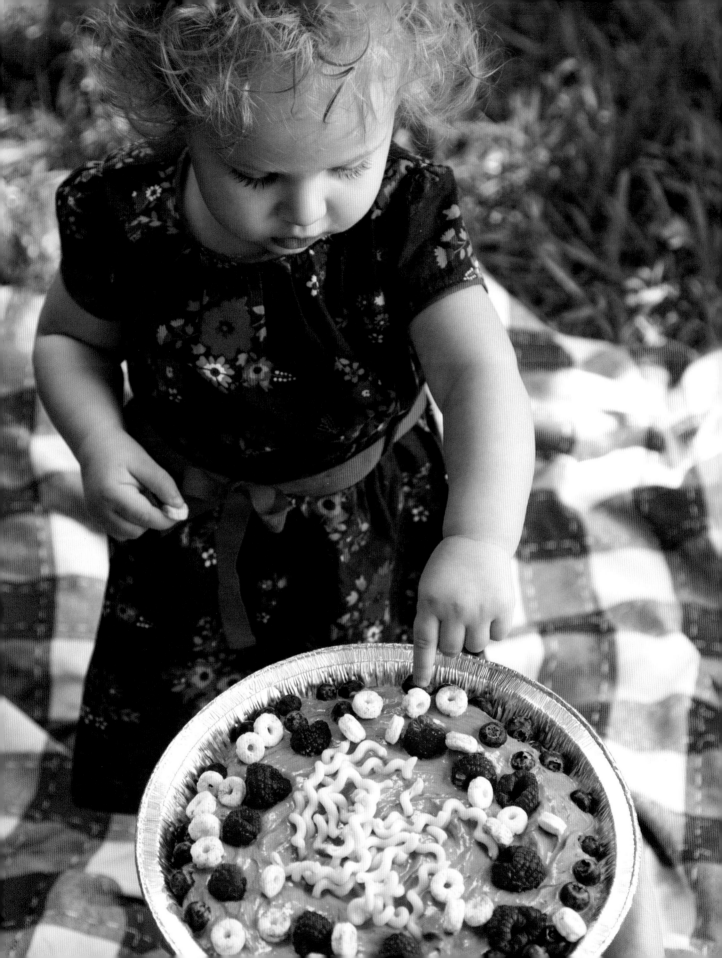

SENSORY PLAY "MUD" PIES

YIELD: *1 big mess*

The combination of still-developing motor skills and an intense curiosity about the world around them gives babies a natural talent for mess making. You can satisfy baby's messy urges and treat that young brain to a unique sensory experience by building a big old mud pie.

INGREDIENTS

» 1 cup (240 ml) plain whole milk yogurt, divided

» 2 tablespoons (30 ml) unsweetened cocoa powder

» ¼ cup (60 ml) fresh raspberries, blueberries, or blackberries

» ¼ cup (60 ml) cereal Os or puffs

» ¼ cup (60 ml) cooked pasta or macaroni

DIRECTIONS

1. Mix the yogurt and cocoa powder together in a small bowl.

2. Place the yogurt and various toppings in small individual bowls suitable for baby (non-breakable).

TO USE

Arrange the bowls of "mud" and toppings within baby's reach. Provide your wee one with a small tin or plastic bowl or pie plate. Encourage baby to build (and taste) a mud pie using the ingredients provided.

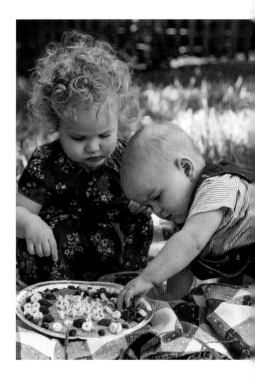

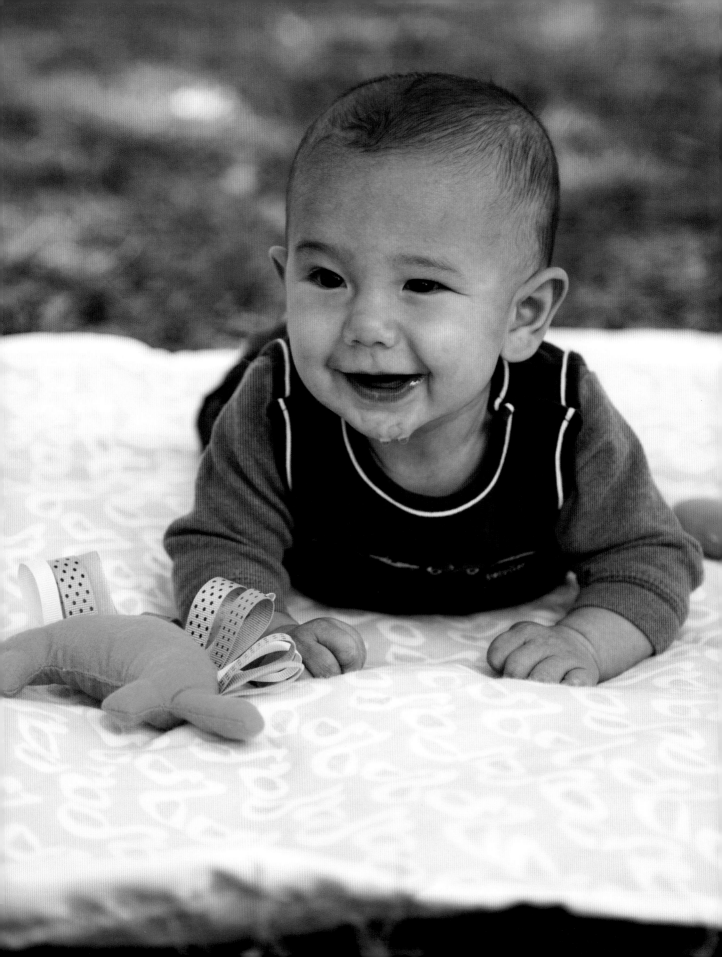

ONE-YARD PLAY MAT

YIELD: *1 play mat*

We all need a soft place to land, and babies are no exception. Fabric play mats give little ones a clean and cozy spot to endure tummy time, practice rolling over, and aim that spittle. As baby grows, the play mat can double as a blanket, super-hero cape, or living room fort topper.

This project makes a perfect gift for expecting parents because it appears far more complicated and time consuming than it actually is. A whole wide world of fabric choices makes customizing play mats as easy as pie, and you can be sure of the item's usefulness. One can never have too many play mats—especially if your child prefers to enjoy tummy time in the buff.

While this project is called a 1-yard play mat, it actually requires 2 yards of fabric and 1 yard of batting—not to mention 3 yards of satin binding. Nevertheless, the mat itself will only be about 1 yard long, and with practice, should take around 1 hour to complete.

MATERIALS + TOOLS

- 1 yard (91cm) flannel or quilter's cotton, first color
- 1 yard (91cm) flannel or quilter's cotton, second color
- 1 yard (91cm) cotton batting
- 3 yards (274cm) extra-wide double-fold bias tape or satin blanket binding
- Matching thread
- Scissors or a rotary cutter with mat
- Sewing machine
- Cereal bowl or other round object
- Safety pins

DIRECTIONS

1. Trim selvage edge from fabric.

2. Place the first piece of fabric right side down on a large flat surface. Place the layer of batting on top, followed by the second piece of fabric, right side up. Trim the batting to match the size of the fabric.

3. Smooth the layered fabric and adjust as needed to make sure that the three pieces line up properly. Insert safety pins into the fabric through all three layers at 6-inch (15cm) intervals in multiple rows (see figure 1, page 174).

4. Use a cereal bowl or other round object to trace round quarter-circles on each corner. Cut round edges off rectangles using the traced shape (see figure 2, page 174).

5. Quilt play mat by stitching straight lines across the play mat between the safety pin rows. Stitch two lines across the short side of the mat and four lines across the long side (see figure 3, page 174).

6. Remove the safety pins.

7. Pin the bias tape or satin binding around the edges of the mat, being careful to line up both sides of the tape evenly. Sew the bias tape onto the mat by stitching close to its top edge (see figure 4, page 174).

8. Turn the mat over and check to see if both sides have been properly stitched. If any sections are still loose, stitch over them again.

ONE-YARD PLAY MAT *(continued)*

Binding   ∂ Safety Pin

Right Side

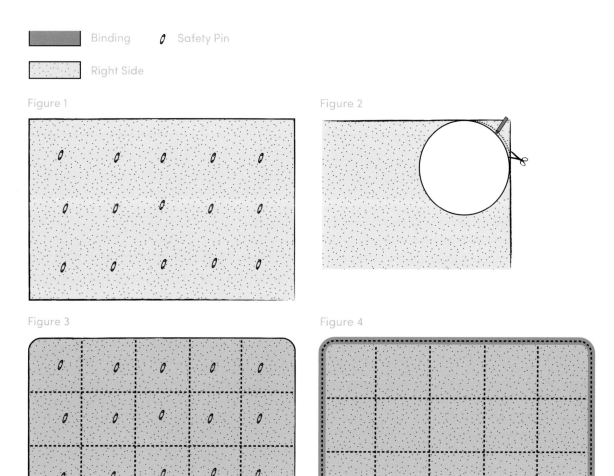

Figure 1

Figure 2

Figure 3

Figure 4

RIBBON SOFTIE

YIELD: *2 ribbon softies*

Babies love to explore new textures. Whether they are using their hands or their mouths, little ones will love squeezing these soft cuddly toys and fiddling with the multicolored ribbons. Add a rattle or squeaker (sources listed on page 194) by stuffing it inside the softie along with the soft fluffy stuffing. Baby will love hearing a fun noise when shaking the toy.

DIRECTIONS

Measure and Cut Pattern Pieces

1. Cut or trace pattern pieces (Ribbon Softie A, Ribbon Softie B) from pattern library (page 188).

2. Fold fabric in half and pin pattern pieces. Cut two of each pattern piece.

3. Cut ribbon into twenty 2-inch (5cm) pieces. To stop the cut ribbon ends from fraying, seal ends with non-toxic fabric glue or melt ends with a heating implement.

Assemble Softies

4. Match up pattern pieces, placing right sides together. Pin edges of each softie carefully, placing extra pins around curves.

5. Insert the ribbons into each softie where indicated by X on the pattern pieces. Pin to secure.

6. Stitch around edges using a ⅛-inch (3mm) seam allowance, leaving a 2-inch (5cm) opening to turn out fabric (see figure 1, page 177).

Finish Softies

7. Turn out each softie (instructions on page 20).

8. Stuff with filling and hand-stitch opening closed (instructions on page 19).

MATERIALS + TOOLS

» ¼ yard (23cm) flannel

» 5 ounces (150 g) loose wool batting or polyester fiberfill

» 1¼ yards (114cm) ribbon in assorted colors

» Non-toxic fabric glue or heating implement

» Matching thread

» Tracing paper and pencil

» Scissors or a rotary cutter with mat

» Pins

» Ruler or measuring tape

» Sewing machine

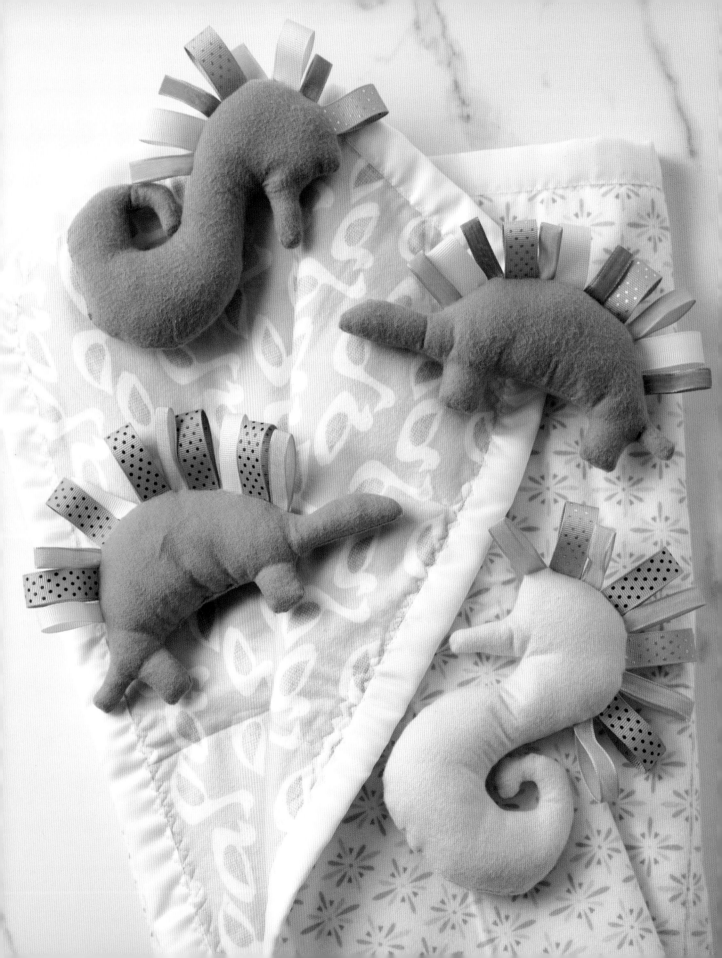

RIBBON SOFTIE *(continued)*

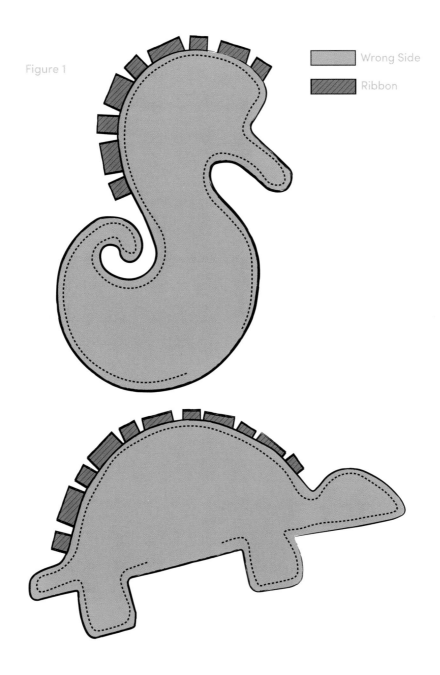

Figure 1

Wrong Side

Ribbon

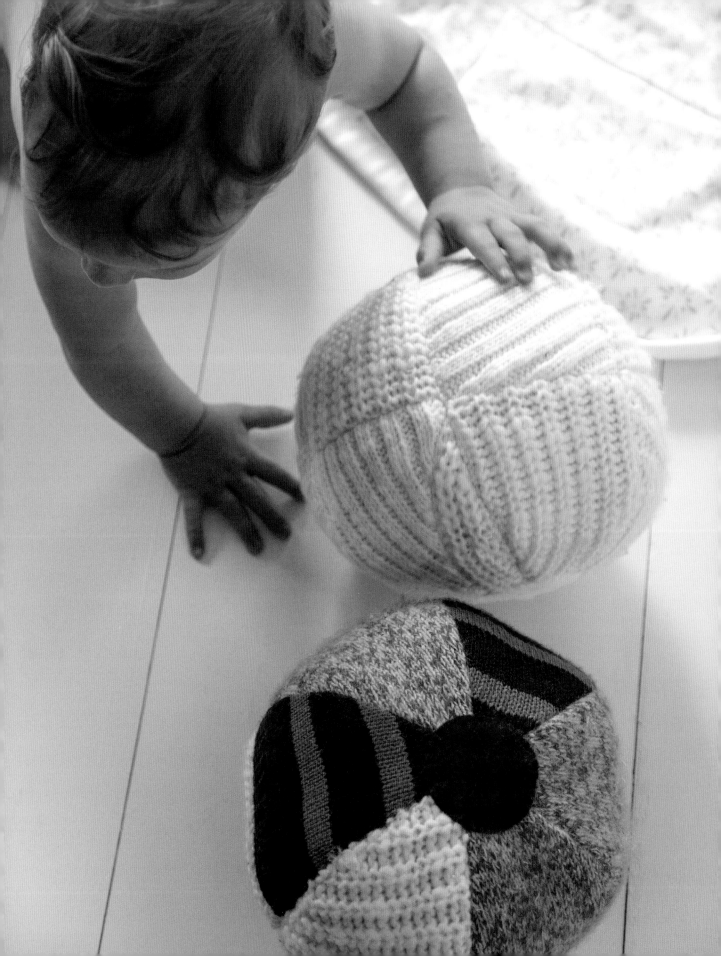

SOFT SWEATER BALL

YIELD: *1 ball*

Large, soft, cuddly playthings like this fuzzy sweater ball are great fun for big and little kids alike. Babies will enjoy tapping and jingling it like a giant rattle, while toddlers can practice rolling, throwing, and chasing it all over the house.

Second-hand sweaters provide a lovely variety of colors and textures for baby to explore, while making use of items that may have otherwise gone to waste. While sweater shopping, look for pieces that are visually appealing and tightly knit. Loose-knit sweaters, like mesh or mohair, will be more difficult to work with. If you'd rather not use sweaters to make your ball, another soft or wooly fabric will do. Wool felt, cotton flannel, or terrycloth would all be great choices.

MATERIALS + TOOLS

- 1 or 2 adult-sized sweaters or ½ yard (46 cm) other soft or wooly fabric)
- ¼ yard (23cm) muslin
- 6 x 6-in. (15 x 15cm) piece wool felt
- 5 ounces (150 g) fiberfill
- 37mm rattle insert
- Tracing paper and pencil
- Ruler or measuring tape
- Chalk or pencil
- Needle and thread
- Pins
- Scissors
- Sewing machine

DIRECTIONS

Deconstruct Sweaters

1. Lay sweaters on flat surface and cut off sleeves and hems. Cut along the seams of the sleeves and body, then turn out flat sections of fabric for cutting pattern pieces.

Measure and Cut Pattern Pieces

2. Measure and cut twelve 5 x 6-inch (12.5 x 12.5cm) rectangles of muslin.

3. Measure and cut twelve 5 x 6-inch (12.5 x 12.5cm) rectangles from sweaters.

4. Cut or trace pattern pieces (Upcycled Sweater Ball A and Upcycled Sweater Ball B) from pattern library (page 190).

5. Trace Upcycled Sweater Ball A pattern onto all twelve muslin pieces with chalk or pencil.

6. Trace Upcycled Sweater Ball B pattern onto wool felt twice. Cut out pattern pieces.

SOFT SWEATER BALL *(continued)*

Assemble Triangle Panels

7. Place sweater pieces right side down with traced muslin on top. Pin together (see figure 1, page 181).

8. Sew layers together by stitching over the traced pattern on the muslin.

9. Trim edges of each panel up to the seam (see figure 2, page 181).

Assemble Ball

10. Match up two triangle panels with right sides together. Sew together on short edge, leaving long sides open. Repeat with remaining panels, making six diamond-shaped pieces (see figure 3, page 181).

11. Match up two diamonds with right sides together. Sew together along one long edge, leaving the other edge open. Repeat with remaining four diamond pieces, making three larger pieces.

12. Match two of the larger pieces with right sides together. Sew together on long edges. Continuing in the same fashion, match the last piece with the assembly and sew together on the long edge, leaving a 2-inch (5cm) opening in the last edge for the project to be turned out and stuffed (see figure 4, page 181).

Finish Ball

13. Turn out project (instructions on page 20).

14. Stuff ball with fiberfill. When ball is about halfway stuffed, place rattle insert inside. Continue stuffing until ball is firmly filled.

15. Hand-stitch the opening closed (instructions on page 19).

16. Pin the wool felt Pattern Piece Bs to top and bottom of ball, covering the spot where the panels all come together. Hand-stitch the pieces onto the ball using the overcast stitch (instructions on page 19); (see figure 5, page 181).

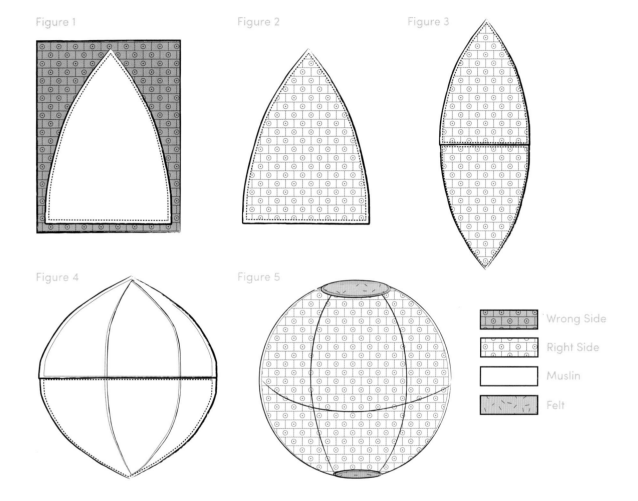

Figure 1

Figure 2

Figure 3

Figure 4

Figure 5

Wrong Side

Right Side

Muslin

Felt

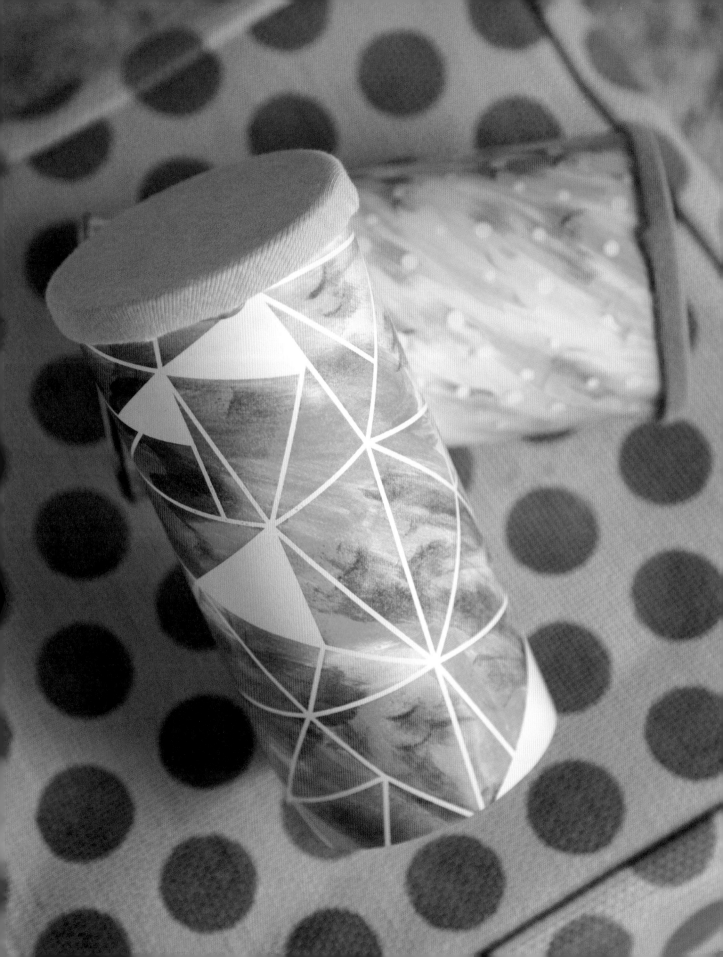

UPCYCLED SHAKERS & DRUMS

YIELD: *1 upcycled shaker*

Kids are easy to please. For them, it's the simple things that make life great—like warm milk, peek-a-boo, and packing materials. The more expensive the toy, the more your baby will love the box that it came in. Children of all ages seem to be fascinated by cardboard boxes, paper canisters, and plastic tubs. Lucky for us, there is no shortage of packaging to keep them busy.

While you could simply hand your little one an empty oatmeal container and make their day, it's sometimes fun to enhance the experience a little. Glue the top back on the canister and now it's a drum. Place a few dried beans or a handful of uncooked rice inside and suddenly it becomes a maraca. The following project utilizes this simple concept to transform an everyday item into a whimsical (and free) toy.

MATERIALS + TOOLS

- 1 empty paperboard canister with lid
- 8 x 8-in. (20 x 20cm) square jersey fabric
- 1 rubber band
- ¼ cup (60 ml) uncooked rice or dried beans
- Decorative paper
- Hot glue gun and glue sticks
- Scissors
- Ruler

DIRECTIONS

1. Clean and dry the paperboard canister and lid thoroughly.

2. Place the fabric down on a flat surface with the lid upside down on top. Pull the fabric toward the center of the lid and secure it with the rubber band. The fabric should be pulled taut, but not so tight that it bends the lid.

3. Measure the height and diameter of the canister, then cut a piece of decorative paper to match those dimensions. Carefully glue the paper to the canister, covering the sides completely.

4. Place rice or beans inside the canister.

5. Cover the top edges (lip) of the canister with hot glue and quickly secure the fabric-covered lid.

6. Allow the glue to cool completely, then test the strength of the lid by giving it a gentle nudge.

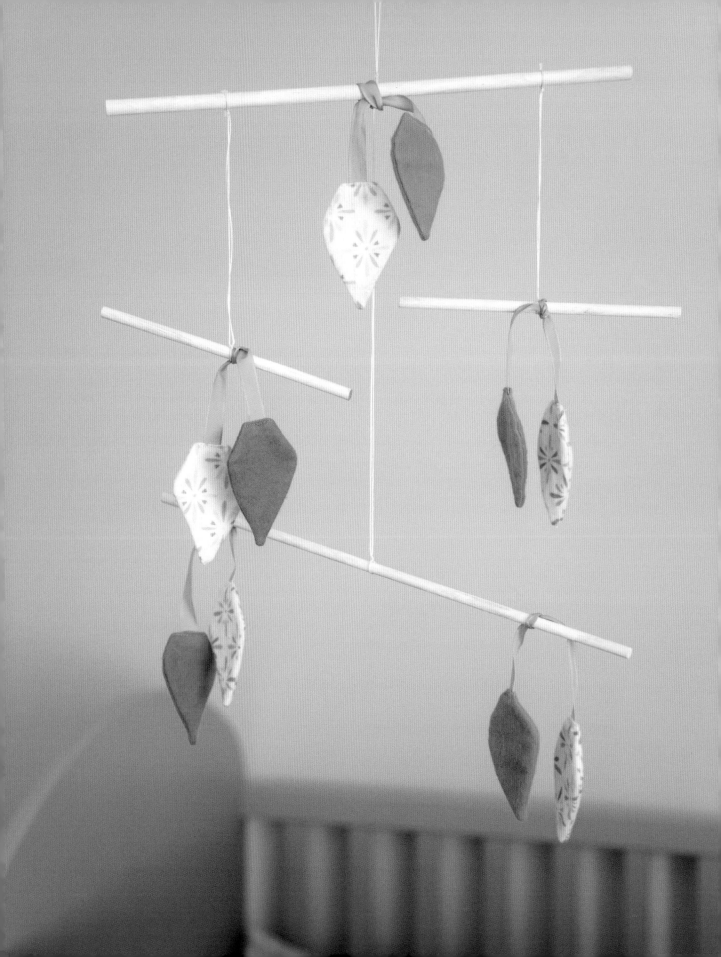

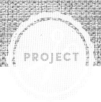
WISHING TREE MOBILE

YIELD: *1 mobile*

The first time I encountered a wishing tree was during a Chinese New Year celebration. The potted tree was covered in tiny ribbons, each with its own handwritten wish scribbled upon it. I remember looking at the tree, shimmering with colored ribbons, and wishing for a baby of my own. Though it was several years before the wish finally came true, I can't help but think of my beautiful son whenever I see a wishing tree.

This project is inspired by wishing trees and the many wishes that we, as parents, have for our children. The idea is for those lovely wishes to stay close to baby through infancy, lovingly displayed in a piece of artwork in the nursery. You can sit down one quiet evening and write your own list of wishes, or ask loved ones to share their own wishes at your baby shower. The tiny handwritten notes will be tucked into the fabric leaves of the mobile before they are stitched up.

MATERIALS + TOOLS

- ¼ yard (23cm) flannel (in assorted colors, if desired)
- 3 yards (274cm) ¼-in. (6mm) ribbon
- 3 feet (91.5cm) ¼-in. (6mm) diameter wooden dowels
- Nylon thread
- Note paper
- White craft paint
- Hot glue gun and glue sticks
- Pen
- Ruler or measuring tape
- Sewing machine
- Scissors

DIRECTIONS

Measure and Cut Pattern and Project Pieces

1. Measure and cut the wooden dowel into two 1-inch (2.5cm) and two 6-inch (15cm) pieces.

2. Measure and cut the ribbon into six 7-inch (18cm) pieces.

3. Measure and cut note paper into twelve 1 x 3-inch (2.5 x 8cm) pieces.

4. Cut or trace the pattern piece (Wishing Tree Mobile) from pattern library (page 190). Cut twenty-four leaves from the flannel.

5. Write wishes on note paper pieces and fold up small enough to fit inside leaves.

6. Paint dowels with white paint and let dry.

WISHING TREE MOBILE *(continued)*

Sew Leaf Pairs

7. Match up leaf pattern pieces into pairs with right sides together. Sew each leaf around edges, leaving the bottom short edge open.

8. Turn out leaves (instructions on page 20).

9. Tuck notes inside leaves.

10. Tuck a ribbon into a leaf and fold leaf edge inside. Stitch opening closed.

11. Tuck other end of ribbon into a second leaf and fold leaf edge inside. Stitch opening closed (see figure 1, right).

12. Repeat last two steps with remaining ribbon and leaves, making six pairs total.

Assemble Mobile

13. Reference figure 2 (at right) throughout these steps. Cut a 20-inch (51cm) piece of thread and fold it in half.

14. Tie the string securely to one long dowel, placing the knot in the exact center of the dowel. Secure thread with a dot of hot glue.

15. Tie a knot in the thread about 7 inches (18cm) from the end. Place the second long dowel in the center of this knot and tie again to hold it firmly in place. Secure with a dot of hot glue.

16. Tie another knot at the end of the thread. This will be the hanger.

17. Cut a 7-inch (18cm) piece of thread and fold it in half.

18. Tie the string securely to one short dowel, placing the knot in the exact center of the dowel. Secure with a dot of hot glue. Repeat with another piece of thread and the second dowel.

19. Tie a knot in each string about 2 inches (5cm) from the end. Tie each of the two short dowels to the top long dowel, placing one on each side, centered between the top string and the ends of the dowel. Secure each with a dot of hot glue.

20. Trim excess thread from mobile.

Decorate Mobile

21. Tie the leaf pairs onto the dowels, spacing them as evenly as possible to keep mobile balanced.

22. Hang mobile from ceiling or high shelf, well away from baby's reach.

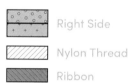

Right Side

Nylon Thread

Ribbon

Figure 1

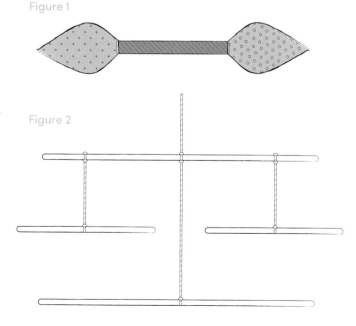

Figure 2

with a song in our hearts

My husband and I both love music. He plays the instruments and I usually sing along. We even had our own little band once upon a time. I always hoped that music would remain a big part of our lives after having children, but I was surprised at how quickly Charlie fell in love with it too. I started singing to him as soon as I got pregnant, and by the time that he was born, had a whole library of lullabies ready to go. As he got older, his father and I began inventing silly songs for everything from changing diapers to watching the dog stroll by. Our family songs have evolved throughout his baby and toddlerhood and now, at two, Charlie adds lines of his own and even invents his own original songs. Whatever you love to do, try sharing it with your children from an early age, then stand back as they take it to places you never imagined!

ASK AN *expert*

Q: What are your favorite kinds of toys for baby's first year?

A: Our son loved anything musical, so we ended up having tons of different-sounding rattles around the house. As he got closer to his first birthday, he demonstrated a love for banging on drums (a love that lives on) and a xylophone he received from a family friend. (Pro tip: Splurge on one that is in tune. You can thank me later.)

—*Sarah Kamalsky, SarahJayn.com*

patterns

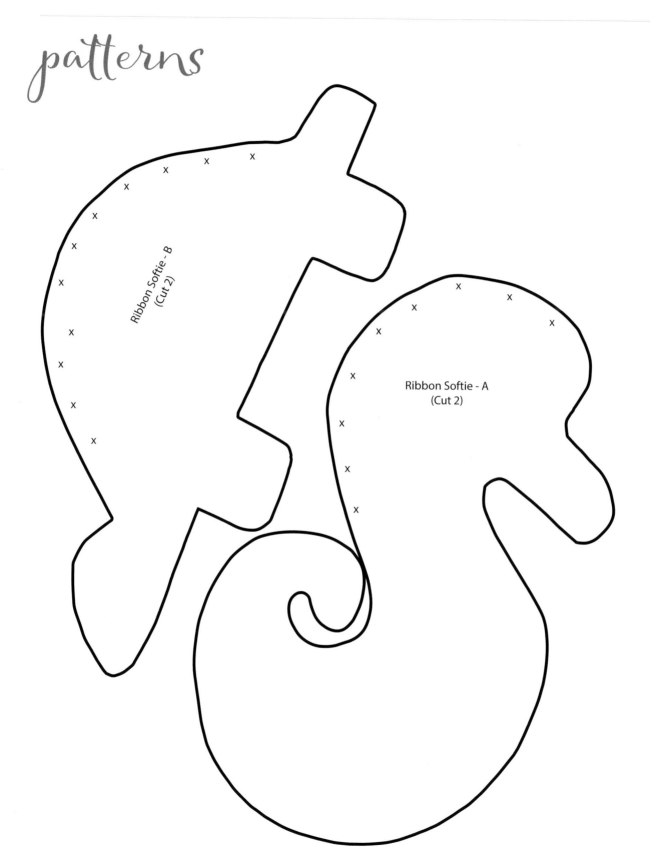

Ribbon Softie - B
(Cut 2)

Ribbon Softie - A
(Cut 2)

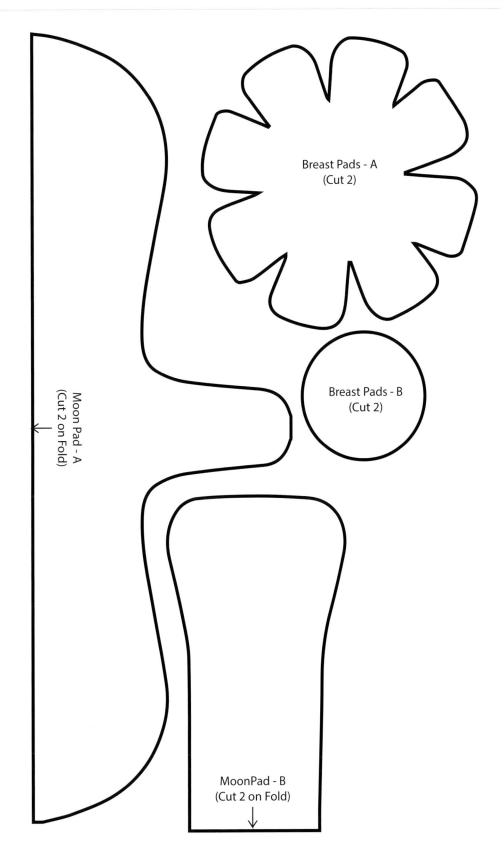

Breast Pads - A
(Cut 2)

Breast Pads - B
(Cut 2)

Moon Pad - A
(Cut 2 on Fold)

MoonPad - B
(Cut 2 on Fold)

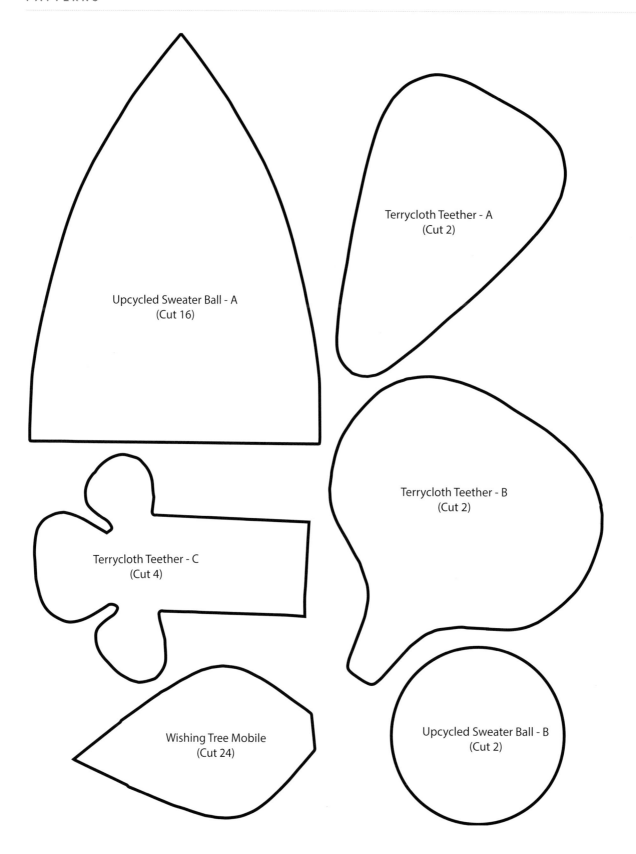

Upcycled Sweater Ball - A
(Cut 16)

Terrycloth Teether - A
(Cut 2)

Terrycloth Teether - B
(Cut 2)

Terrycloth Teether - C
(Cut 4)

Wishing Tree Mobile
(Cut 24)

Upcycled Sweater Ball - B
(Cut 2)

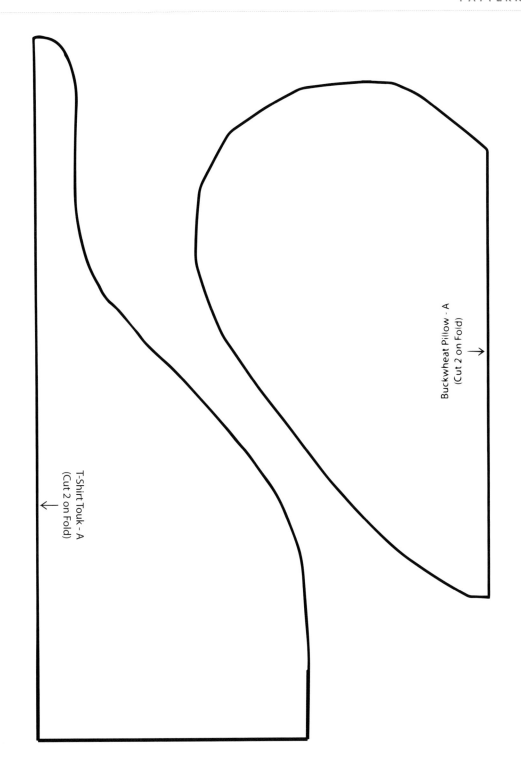

Buckwheat Pillow - A
(Cut 2 on Fold)

T-Shirt Touk - A
(Cut 2 on Fold)

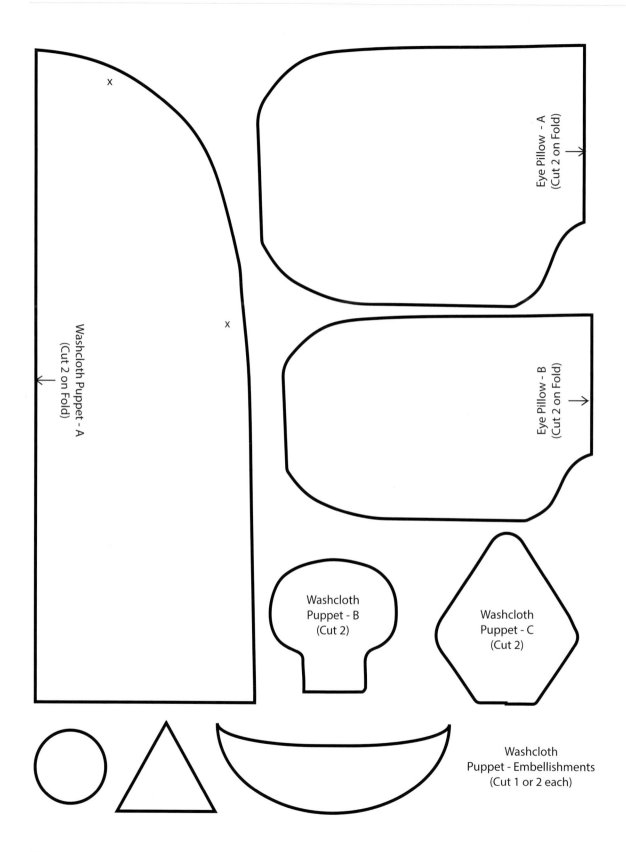

Eye Pillow - A
(Cut 2 on Fold)

Eye Pillow - B
(Cut 2 on Fold)

Washcloth Puppet - A
(Cut 2 on Fold)

Washcloth
Puppet - B
(Cut 2)

Washcloth
Puppet - C
(Cut 2)

Washcloth
Puppet - Embellishments
(Cut 1 or 2 each)

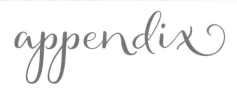

appendix

resources

BABY GEAR AND DIAPERING

Baby Earth
Gear and supplies for diapering, feeding, bath and body, babywearing, and more
babyearth.com

Enlightened Baby
Mindful gear for mama, baby, and tots
enlightenedbaby.com

Fluff Love University
Information on cloth diapering
fluffloveuniversity.com

The Natural Baby Company
Gear and supplies for diapering, feeding, bath and body, babywearing, and more
thenaturalbabyco.com

BREAST-FEEDING SUPPORT

La Leche League
Nursing support groups, education, resources, and online community
llli.org

International Lactation Consultant Association
Lactation consultant directory
ilca.org/why-ibclc/falc

FAVORITE BLOGS AND INFORMATIONAL WEB SITES

Celebration Nutrition
Online nutritional counseling and meal planning services
celebrationnutrition.com

Cool Mom Eats
Family-focused recipes, meal ideas, and more
eats.coolmompicks.com

Cool Mom Picks
Product reviews and recommendations from real moms
Coolmompicks.com

Cookistry
Recipes from cookbook author Donna Currie
cookistry.com

Great Moments in Parenting
Stories from the agony and ecstasy of life with kids
greatmomentsinparenting.com

Hello Glow
Healthy recipes, skin care, and craft projects with a green focus
helloglow.co

Hilah Cooking
Easy recipes and fun cooking videos from Hilah Johnson
hilahcooking.com

Jennifer Pierce Health
Holistic health coaching, recipes, and online detox programs
jenniferpiercehealth.com

Kelly Mom
Educational articles on pregnancy, baby care, breast-feeding, and parenting
kellymom.com

Mama Natural
Crunchy parenting tips, natural pregnancy info, and more
mamanatural.com

Mary Makes Good
My own personal blog, which features DIY beauty recipes, as well as recipes and projects for the home, kitchen, and family
marymakesgood.com

Mommypotamus
Natural health, remedies, and DIY
mommypotamus.com

Mother Rising
A holistic pregnancy blog
motherrisingbirth.com

Natural Beauty Workshop
A natural beauty blog owned by the cosmetic ingredient supplier From Nature with Love. This site features hundreds of free recipes, detailed ingredient information, and more. Authored by yours truly!
naturalbeautyworkshop.com

The National Association for Holistic Aromatherapy (NAHA)
Essential oil safety
naha.org

Wellness Mama
Home remedies, healthy recipes, and DIY
wellnessmama.com

FURTHER READING ON INGREDIENT TOXICITY IN CONSUMER PRODUCTS

Environmental Working Group
A leading resource for information on product safety, EWG's site features tools and articles to help you shop more safely for home and personal care products. The site also includes links to research and articles on why certain ingredients are considered unsafe.
ewg.org

Environmental Working Group's Skin Deep Cosmetics Database
The EWG has done an amazing job of compiling scientific data on almost any ingredient you might find in commercial home and personal care products. You can search Skin Deep's Web site or smart phone app by ingredient or by product to view ingredient information and safety ratings.
ewg.org/skindeep

Campaign for Safe Cosmetics
Learn more about dangerous additives and ingredients used in cosmetics and how you can help join the fight to ban harmful substances from personal care products.
safecosmetics.org

Consumer Safety
Product safety guides, alerts, and news
consumersafety.org

Organic Consumer's Association
A great resource for learning more about the personal and ecological safety of consumer products. The Organic Consumer's Association focuses on campaigning for safer, more sustainable food, cosmetics, and consumer goods.
organicconsumers.org

HEALTH FOOD AND NATURAL HOME CARE

Bob's Red Mill
Specialty grains, flours, and baking ingredients
bobsredmill.com/shop.html

India Tree
Natural food dyes and baking supplies
indiatree.com

Mighty Nest
Eco-friendly products for home, kitchen, and baby care
mightynest.com

LOCAL COMMUNITY SUPPORT

Baby Boot Camp
Nationwide organization offering mom and mom and baby workout sessions
babybootcamp.com

Babywearing International
Worldwide organization sharing babywearing education, meetups, and gear-lending libraries
babywearinginternational.org

Care Calendar
Free care and meal planning calendar for family and friends
carecalendar.org

City Moms Blog Network
A network of city-specific blogs, events, meetups, and online forums
citymomsblog.com

Fit 4 Mom
Nationwide organization offering mom and mom-and-baby workout sessions
fit4mom.com

Hike It Baby
Nationwide organization hosting family hikes
hikeitbaby.com

Meal Train
Free care and meal planning calendar for family and friends
mealtrain.com

Meetup
Directory of local meeting groups for a wide range of topics including moms and kids
meetup.com

ParentAbility
Local breast-feeding support, mom's groups, and parenting workshops based in Austin, TX
tanjaknutson.com

SUPPLIES FOR DIY SKIN CARE

From Nature with Love
Wholesale supplier of 1,750+ natural and complementary ingredients used in skin care, hair care, and soap making. This is a great source for oils, butters, essential oils, hydrosols, exfoliants, clays, and packaging.
fromnaturewithlove.com

Mountain Rose Herbs
Another good resource for basic ingredients, as well as finished natural products
mountainroseherbs.com

Vermont Soap
All-natural cold processed bar and liquid castile soaps
vermontsoap.com

SUPPLIES FOR SEWING AND CRAFTS

You can also find sewing and crafts supplies at your local fabric or crafts store.

American Felt and Craft
Felt, notions, sewing kits, and rattle inserts
feltandcraft.com

Honey Be Good Fabric
Online fabric store offering a wide selection of natural and organic fabric, thread, and batting
honeybegood.com

Lemon Tree Supplies
Sewing supplies, notions, and rattle inserts
lemontree.etsy.com

Organic Cotton Plus
Organic and natural fabrics, notions, and sewing supplies
organiccottonplus.com

Spoonflower
Enormous selection of print fabrics made from indie artist designs or custom printed to order
spoonflower.com

While She Naps
Softie sewing patterns, supplies, and rattle inserts
whileshenaps.etsy.com

endnotes

[1] **International Federation of Professional Aromatherapists,** *IFPA Pregnancy Guidelines,* http://naha.org/assets/uploads/PregnancyGuidelines-Oct11.pdf

[2] **National Institute of Health, Office of Dietary Supplements.** *Health Information for Health Professionals,* https://ods.od.nih.gov/factsheets/list-all/

[2] **Mahan LK, Escott-Stump S, Raymond JL.** *Krause's Food and the Nutrition Care Process* (13th ed). (St. Louis, MO: Elsevier, Inc., 2012.)

contributors

STACIE BILLIS
Food Editor & Cookbook Author
eats.coolmompicks.com

Stacie Billis is a mom of two, the author of *Make It Easy: 120 Mix-and-Match Recipes to Cook from Scratch—with Smart Store-Bought Shortcuts When You Need Them,* and the managing editor of CoolMomEats.com. A leading voice in the conversation about family eating, Stacie brings a unique perspective thanks to her MA in Child Development from Teacher's College, Columbia University. And her non-judgy approach to feeding kids does not preclude an occasional spoonful of Nutella.

DONNA CURRIE
Cookistry
cookistry.com

Donna Currie is a Colorado blogger who has not one, but three different blogs. Cookistry focuses on recipes, Cookistry Reviews is all about cooking-related gadgets and edibles, and Munching on Books is a book review blog that's not quite all cookbooks. Donna also is the author of the cookbook *Make Ahead Bread.*

STEPHANIE L. DARBY, RD, LD
Celebration Nutrition LLC
celebrationnutrition.com

Stephanie is a registered and licensed dietitian based in Austin, Texas. After seeing friends struggle to figure out confusing medically prescribed diets, she started Celebration Nutrition, a private practice that helps individuals with specialized dietary needs find the joy in food and celebrate healthy, full lives. As an avid cook, blogger, and runner, Stephanie spends her free time in the kitchen, creating healthy plant-based recipes for friends and family.

HILAH JOHNSON
Hilah Cooking
HilahCooking.com

Hilah Johnson started HilahCooking.com in 2010 with her husband, Christopher Sharpe. Since then, they've published more than 500 how-to videos and five cookbooks. Hilah has been called everything from "hilarious" to "trashy," which just shows that funny is in the eye of the beholder.

SARAH KAMALSKY
Textile Artist
sarahjayn.com

Sarah Jayn Kamalsky is a daydreaming textile artist and fiber arts fanatic living in Austin, Texas. You can follow her misadventures as a stay-at-home, work-at-home, kinda-maybe-homeschool mom at her blog.

SARA KLEINSMITH
Yoga Instructor
sarakleinsmith.com

Sara Kleinsmith is a yoga teacher, writer, and mom living in Austin, Texas. Her writing has appeared in YogaDork, Scary Mommy, Thought Catalog, and Elephant Journal. Sara is a lover of embodied anatomy and loves working with new moms and yogaphobes.

TANJA KNUTSON, IBCLC
ParentAbility
tanjaknutson.com

Tanja Knutson is a Parenting Coach and an International Board-Certified Lactation Consultant (IBCLC) working both in private practice and in hospital. She lives in the Austin, Texas area with her husband, four children, and multiple furry rescues. She is the founder of ParentAbility, which guides parents through all the steep learning curves of parenthood, starting with prenatal breast-feeding classes, lactation home visits, new moms' groups, and parenting workshops called How to Talk So Kids Will Listen.

Since 2001, she has volunteered with La Leche League International as a Leader and District Coordinator (Asia). She credits La Leche League with helping her overcome her own breast-feeding challenges, listen to her heart, and find her calling: guiding women as they learn mothering.

Having lived and worked in four countries, Tanja sees that mothers around the world often face the same fundamental concerns: how to be a good parent and raise a healthy baby. She firmly believes that "it takes a village to raise a parent" and is committed to building connected communities where parents feel supported—with kindness and compassion—as they grow into their roles.

JENNIFER PIERCE
Holistic Health Coach
JenniferPierceHealth.com

Jennifer Pierce is a certified holistic health coach, wellness advocate, yoga instructor, food and travel blogger, recovering CPA, and green smoothie junkie. When she is not working and blogging, you can find her hiking the greenbelt, attending or teaching a sweaty yoga session, hanging out with her nieces, enjoying the live music scene in Austin, and planning her next travel adventure.

DR. SUZANNE VAN BENTHUYSEN, MD, FAAP, IBCLC
Bee Well Pediatrics
beewellaustin.com

Dr. Suzanne Van Benthuysen is an integrative pediatrician and board-certified lactation consultant in Austin, Texas. She enjoys working with mothers to meet their breast-feeding goals and providing families with evidence-based complementary and alternative medication treatment options.

index

Note: Page numbers in italics indicate recipes and projects; page numbers in bold indicate contributor biographical sketches and contact information; and page numbers in parentheses indicate patterns.

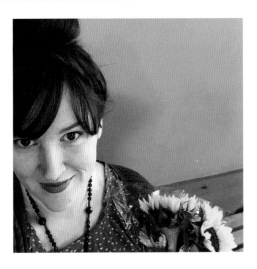

about the author

Mary Helen Leonard is a natural lifestyle writer and educator living in Austin, Texas. She has spent ten years working in the natural skin care industry, formulating do-it-yourself recipes for the popular natural skin care blog, www.NaturalBeautyWorkshop.com. Mary Helen also writes about food, family, and DIY at www.MaryMakesGood.com. When she's not in the kitchen whipping something up you can find her snapping photos, sewing freestyle quilts, or snuggling up to her son, Charlie.

MORE GREAT BOOKS *from*
SPRING HOUSE PRESS

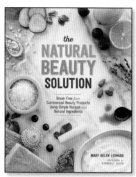
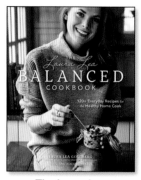
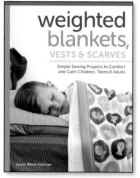
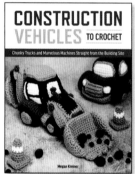
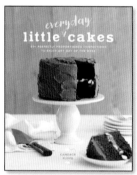
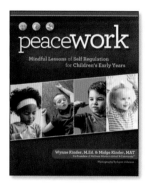
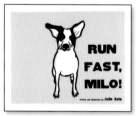
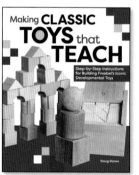
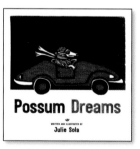